OXFORD PSYCH

D1766086

ADHD and Hyperkinetic Disorder

by

Tobias Banaschewski

David Coghill

Marina Danckaerts

Manfred Döpfner

Luis Rohde

Joseph A. Sergeant

Edmund J.S. Sonuga-Barke

Eric Taylor

Alessandro Zuddas

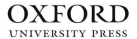

OXFORD
UNIVERSITY PRESS

OXFORD
UNIVERSITY PRESS

Great Clarendon Street, Oxford OX2 6DP

Oxford University Press is a department of the University of Oxford.
It furthers the University's objective of excellence in research, scholarship,
and education by publishing worldwide in

Oxford New York

Auckland Cape Town Dar es Salaam Hong Kong Karachi
Kuala Lumpur Madrid Melbourne Mexico City Nairobi
New Delhi Shanghai Taipei Toronto

With offices in

Argentina Austria Brazil Chile Czech Republic France Greece
Guatemala Hungary Italy Japan Poland Portugal Singapore
South Korea Switzerland Thailand Turkey Ukraine Vietnam

Oxford is a registered trade mark of Oxford University Press
in the UK and in certain other countries

Published in the United States
by Oxford University Press Inc., New York

British Library Cataloguing in Publication Data

Data available

Library of Congress Cataloging in Publication Data

Data available

Typeset by Newgen Imaging Systems (P) Ltd., Chennai, India
Printed in Great Britain
on acid-free paper by
Ashford Colour Press Ltd., Gosport, Hampshire.

ISBN 978-0-19-957765-1

10 9 8 7 6 5 4 3 2 1

Contents

Contributors *vii*

Abbreviations list *ix*

1 Introduction
  Eric Taylor   1

2 Phenomenology
  Tobias Banaschewski and Luis Rohde   3

3 Pathogenesis
  Edmund Sonuga-Barke   19

4 Assessment
  David Coghill and Joseph A. Sergeant   33

5 Pharmacological treatments
  Alessandro Zuddas   53

6 Psychosocial and other non-pharmacological
  treatments
  Manfred Döpfner   77

7 Organizing and delivering treatment
  David Coghill and Marina Danckaerts   91

8 Appendix   107

Index *115*

Contributors

Tobias Banaschewski
Professor
University of Heidelberg,
Director
Department of Child
and Adolescent Psychiatry,
Central Institute
of Mental Health,
Mannheim, Germany

David Coghill
Senior Lecturer
Department of Psychiatry,
University of Dundee,
Dundee, UK

Marina Danckaerts
Professor Katholieke
Universiteit Leuven,
Department of Child and
Adolescent Psychiatry,
University Hospital Leuven,
Belgium

Manfred Döpfner
Professor
Departments of Psychiatry and
Psychotherapy of Childhood
and Adolescence,
University of Cologne/Köln,
Köln, Germany

Luis Rohde
Professor
Child and Adolescent
Psychiatric Division,
Hospital de Clinicas de Porto
Alegre,
Porto Alegre, Brazil

Joseph A. Sergeant
Professor
Department of Clinical
Neuropsychology,
Faculty of Psychology
and Education,
Vrije Universitat,
Amsterdam, the Netherlands

Edmund J.S. Sonuga-Barke
Professor
Department of Psychology,
University of Southampton,
Southampton, UK

Eric Taylor
Professor
Department of Child &
Adolescent Psychiatry,
Institute of Psychiatry,
Kings College London,
London, UK

Alessandro Zuddas
Associate Professor
of Child Neuropsychiatry,
Department of Neuroscience,
University of Cagliari,
Cagliari, Italy

Abbreviations list

5-HTTLPR	serotonin transporter gene, polymorphisms within the promoter region
ADHD	attention deficit hyperactivity disorder
ADHD-RS	ADHD Rating Scale
ADORE	Attention Deficit Hyperactivity Disorder Observational Research in Europe
AERS	Adverse Event Reporting System
APA	American Psychiatric Association
ATX	atomoxetine
BASC	Behavioural Assessment System for Children
BID	twice daily
BPT	behavioural parent training
BPVS	British Picture Vocabulary Scale
CAI	computer assisted instruction
CAMHS	Child and Adolescent Mental Health Service
CANTAB	Cambridge Neuropsychological Test Automated Battery
CAPA	Child and Adolescent Psychiatric Assessment
CBCL	Child Behaviour Checklist
CBF	cerebral blood flow
CBT	cognitive-behaviour therapy
CD	conduct disorder
CDI	Child Depression Inventory
CGAS	Children's Global Assessment Scale
CGI-I	Clinical Global Impression Improvement Scale
CGI-S	Clinical Global Impression Severity Scale
CHIP-CE	Child Health and Illness Profile Child Edition
CHMP	European Medicines Agency (EMEA)'s Committee for Medicinal Products for Human Use
CPRS-R	Conners Parent Rating Scale - Revised
CPT	Continuous Performance Test

CPT MRT	Continuous Performance Test Mean Reaction Time
CSBQ	Children's Social Behaviour Questionnaire
CSHQ	Children's Sleep Habits Questionnaire
CTRS-R	Conners Teacher Rating Scales - Revised
CWPT	classwide peer tutoring
CYP2D6	cytochrome P450 2D6 enzymatic system
DA	dopamine
DAT1	dopamine transporter
DAWBA	Development and Well-being Assessment
DCD-Q	Developmental Coordination Disorder Questionnaire
DHA	docosahexaenoic acid
DHPG	3,4-dihydroxyphenylethylene glycol
DICA	Diagnostic Interview for Children and Adolescents
DISC	Diagnostic Interview Schedule for Children
DISC-IV	Diagnostic Interview Schedule for Children based on DSM-IV
DNA	Desoxyribonuclein acid
DRD4	dopamine D4 receptor
DSM-III	Diagnostic and Statistical Manual of Mental Disorders, third edition
DSM-III-R	Diagnostic and Statistical Manual of Mental Disorders, third edition, revised version
DSM-IV	Diagnostic and Statistical Manual of Mental Disorders, fourth edition
ECG	electrocardiogram
EEG	electroencephalogram
EF	executive functions
EPA	eicosapentaenoic acid
ERPs	event-related potentials
EUNETHYDIS	European Network for Hyperkinetic Disorders
F-A-S	Fluency Test; Version of the Controlled Oral Word Association Test using the letters F, A, and S
FDA	US Food and Drug Administration
FISH	fluorescence in-situ hybridization
GH	growth hormone
HKD	hyperkinetic disorder

ICD-10	International Classification of Diseases, 10th revision
IR	immediate release
K-SADS-PL	Schedule for Affective Disorders and Schizophrenia for School-age Children
MAO	monoamine oxidase
MPH	methylphenidate
MRI	Magnetic Resonance Imaging
MTA	Multimodal Treatment Study of ADHD
NE	norepinephrine
NET	norepinephrine transporter
NICE	National Institute for Health and Clinical Excellence
NNT	Numbers Needed to Treat
OCD	obsessive compulsive disorder
ODD	oppositional defiant disorder
PACS	Parental Account of Children's Symptoms
PATS	Preschoolers with ADHD Treatment Study
PD	pharmacodynamic
PDD	pervasive developmental disorder
PEDS-QL	Pediatric Quality of Life Inventory
PET	Positron Emission Tomography
PK	pharmacokinetics
P-YMRS	Parent version of the Young Mania Rating Scale
R-CMAS	Revised Children's Manifest Anxiety Scale
RCT	Randomized Controlled Trial
SCQ	Social Communication Questionnaire
SDQ	Strengths and Difficulties Questionnaire
SERT	serotonin transporter
SIGN	Scottish Intercollegiate Guidelines Network
SKAMP	Swanson, Kotkin, Atkins, McFlynn & Pelham Scale
SMD	standardized mean difference
SNAP	Swanson, Nolan and Pelham Questionnaire
SNAP-IV	Swanson, Nolan and Pelham Questionnaire, revised DSM-IV version
SPECT	Single Photon Emission Computed Tomography
SSRI	selective serotonin reuptake inhibitors
SSRT	Stop Signal Reaction Time

SWAN	Strengths and Weaknesses of ADHD—Symptoms and Normal Behavior
TEACH	Test of Every Day Attention of Children
TOWRE	Test of Word Reading Efficiency
Trails B	Trail Making Test B
TRF	Teacher Rating Form
VMAT-2	Vesicular Monoamine Transporter 2
WAIS	Wechsler Adult Intelligence Scale
WASI	Wechsler Abbreviated Scale of Intelligence
WCST	Wisconsin Card Sorting Test
WHO	World Health Organization
WISC	Wechsler Intelligence Scale for Children
WISC III	Wechsler Intelligence Scale for Children, Third Edition
WM	working memory
Y-BOCS	Yale-Brown Obsessive Compulsive Scale

Chapter 1

Introduction

Eric Taylor

Hyperkinetic disorder and ADHD matter—as conditions making risks for poor mental health later; as a focus of controversy about the rights and wrongs of psychopathological approaches; and as treatable disorders that are often untreated.

European psychiatry tended to avoid the diagnosis until the 1990s, or even to regard "ADHD" as an American aberration. The last decade, however, has seen a major increase in practice and research. Specialist assessments are much more widely available; diagnosis and drug treatment are better understood and better provided.

Increasing knowledge has created new needs for practice. Child psychiatrists, for example, need a wide range of skills in accurate and safe prescribing of the increasing range of effective psychotropic drugs. Primary medical care needs to know how to recognize the condition, as well as when to refer to a specialist.

Paediatricians will need a good understanding of the advances that have taken place in psychological treatment, and therefore of the range of non-medical interventions that should now be provided.

Clinical psychologists need to draw on the advancing knowledge about the neuropsychological foundations in order to enrich treatment programmes.

Adult psychiatrists will often need a guide to the recognition and treatment of conditions characterized by inattentiveness and impulsiveness—many such cases have until recently been regarded simply as parts of personality disorder (or atypical bipolar disorder).

Teachers and remedial education specialists will need a fuller understanding of how many "maladjusted" children can be helped by recognizing their inattentiveness and impulsiveness as targets for intervention.

All groups should be able to profit from an understanding of the changes that are at the heart of the disorder, so that they can convey the understanding to the people affected by the disorder. The problems of hyperkinesis are not only for the sufferer—they extend to parents and siblings, to classmates and teachers, to employers and employees.

The authors of this book have been at the forefront of clinical science. They are unified by membership of a European network, EUNETHYDIS, led by Professor Sergeant. The network has enabled them to meet together, to make systematic and critical reviews of the international literature, to develop published guidelines, and to join basic scientists in multi-centre genetic and neuropsychological research.

This book provides a concise and authoritative account of modern knowledge about hyperkinetic disorder and ADHD. It is recommended to all those who need to know about them.

Chapter 2

Phenomenology

Tobias Banaschewski and Luis Rohde

Key points

- The core symptoms of ADHD are inattention, hyperactivity, and impulsivity
- As the presentation and challenges of ADHD change over time, clinicians must take a lifespan approach and follow patients closely, modifying their care and treatment according to the individual's current needs
- Comorbid conditions are the rule in clinical samples
- ADHD is associated with seriously impairment for patient, family and society.

2.1 Definitions

Attention-Deficit/Hyperactivity Disorder (ADHD) and Hyperkinetic Disorder (HKD) are defined as psychiatric disorders characterized by a developmentally inappropriate, pervasive (across different situations such as home and school) and persistent pattern of severe inattention, hyperactivity, and/or impulsivity with an onset in early childhood that is associated with substantial impairment in social, academic and/or occupational functioning.

Both diagnoses, ADHD (DSM-IV, American Psychiatric Association, 1994, 2000) and HKD (ICD-10, WHO, 1992) are based upon the almost identical sets of 18 symptoms (Table 2.1). However, there are major differences in the decision rules determining that HKD is a subset of ADHD in ICD-10 and can be used to identify a more restricted and refined phenotype, which is accompanied more impairment and inhibitory control deficits and which does imply a slightly different treatment algorithm (Swanson *et al.*, 1998; Taylor *et al.*, 2004; Schachar *et al.*, 2007; see also Chapter 5–7).

Box 2.1 ADHD/HKD: Core symptoms

The core symptoms are:

- Inattention
- Impulsivity and
- Hyperactivity

These symptoms are required to be:

- present from an early age (before the age of 6 (ICD-10) or 7 years (DSM-IV)),
- pervasive across at least 2 situations (e.g. home, school, and social life) and
- the cause of significant impairment to functioning.

Table 2.1 Symptom domains for ADHD/HKD in DSM-IV & ICD-10

Inattention

Often ...

- fails to give close attention to detail or makes careless mistakes in schoolwork, work, or other activities
- has difficulty sustaining attention in tasks or play activities
- does not seem to listen when spoken to directly
- does not follow through on instructions and fails to finish schoolwork, chores, or duties in the workplace (not due to oppositional behaviour or failure to understand instructions)
- has difficulty organizing tasks and activities
- avoids, dislikes, or is reluctant to engage in tasks that require sustained mental effort (such as schoolwork or homework)
- loses things necessary for tasks or activities (e.g., toys, school assignments, pencils, books, or tools)
- easily distracted by extraneous stimuli
- forgetful in daily activities.

Hyperactivity

Often ...

- fidgets with hands or feet or squirms in seat
- leaves seat in classroom or in other situations in which remaining seated is expected
- runs about or climbs excessively in situations in which it is inappropriate (in adolescents or adults, may be limited to subjective feelings of restlessness)
- has difficulty playing or engaging in leisure activities quietly
- 'on the go' or often acts as if 'driven by a motor' (DSM-IV); exhibits a persistent pattern of excessive motor activity that is not substantially modified by social context or demands (ICD-10)
- talks excessively (DSM-IV).

Impulsivity

Often ...

- talks excessively without appropriate response to social constraints (ICD-10)
- blurts out answers before questions have been completed
- has difficulty awaiting turn in games or group situations
- interrupts or intrudes on others (e.g., butts into conversations or games).

DSM-IV lists 18 symptoms covering 2 dimensions: inattention and hyperactivity/impulsivity. It distinguishes 3 clinical subtypes of ADHD: a predominantly inattentive subtype, which displays at least 6 (or more) symptoms of inattention and less than 6 of hyperactivity/impulsivity, a predominantly hyperactive/impulsive subtype suffering from 6 (or more) symptoms of hyperactivity-impulsivity and less than 6 of inattention, and a combined subtype, which meets both sets of criteria (see Box 2.1).

The symptoms must have persisted for at least 6 months, must occur pervasively across at least 2 situations (e.g. home, school and social life), and some of them must have been present causing impairment before 7 years of age. Furthermore, these symptoms are required to not occur exclusively during the course of a pervasive developmental disorder, schizophrenia, or other psychotic disorder and not to be better accounted for by another mental disorder. DSM-IV diagnostic criteria for ADHD are outlined in Table 2.2.

Although the ICD-10 criteria for hyperkinetic disorder describe similar symptoms to DSM-IV, ICD-10 criteria are more restrictive in that they require:

- Hyperactivity, impulsivity, and inattention all to be present (in addition to at least 6 inattention symptoms, the presence of at least 3 hyperactive symptoms and at least 1 impulsive symptom)
- All symptoms to be impairing across two or more settings
- An exclusion of the diagnosis if mania, depression, and/or anxiety disorders are also present, whereas DSM-IV allows these diagnoses to be made as comorbid conditions (see Table 2.3).

Table 2.2 DSM-IV diagnostic criteria for ADHD

A Either 1 or 2

1 Six (or more) of symptoms of inattention have persisted for at least 6 months to a degree that is maladaptive and inconsistent with developmental level.

2 Six (or more) of symptoms of hyperactivity-impulsivity have persisted for at least 6 months to a degree that is maladaptive and inconsistent with developmental level.

B Some hyperactive-impulsive or inattentive symptoms that caused impairment were present before 7 years of age.

C Some impairment from the symptoms is present in 2 or more settings (e.g., at school [or work] or at home).

D There must be clear evidence of clinically significant impairment in social, academic, or occupational functioning.

E The symptoms do not occur exclusively during the course of a pervasive developmental disorder, schizophrenia, or other psychotic disorder and are not better accounted for by another mental disorder (e.g., mood disorder, anxiety disorder, dissociative disorder, or personality disorder).

The application of these more restrictive criteria defines as hyperkinetic disorder the subgroup of those patients with combined type ADHD with the most severely impairing symptomatology. The main subdivision is between HKD and Hyperkinetic Conduct Disorder, the latter defining a category of HKD plus conduct disorder.

Both classification systems include a criterion for the age of onset of symptoms causing impairment (before the age of 6 (ICD-10), respectively seven years (DSM-IV)). However, this criterion's clinical validity is currently not supported by scientific evidence. It is recommended that clinicians do not rule out the possibility of a diagnosis of ADHD in patients who have not had symptoms causing impairment before the age of 7 years.

Table 2.3 Differences between DSM-IV and ICD-10 criteria of ADHD or HKD		
	DSM-IV ADHD	**ICD-10 HKD**
Symptoms	Either or both of following: • At least 6 of 9 inattentive symptoms • At least 6 of 9 hyperactive or impulsive symptoms	All of following: • At least 6 of 8 inattentive symptoms • At least 3 of 5 hyperactive symptoms • At least 1 of 4 impulsive symptoms
Cross-Situational Pervasiveness	Some impairment from symptoms is present in more than one setting such as home and school	Criteria are met for more than one setting such as home and school
Age of onset	Some symptoms that cause impairment are present before age 7 years	Symptoms should be present before age 6 years
Comorbid Diagnoses	Comorbid diagnosis with conduct, anxiety, and mood disorders recommended if inclusion criteria of multiple disorders are met	Diagnosis of HKD if there are anxiety and mood disorders is not recommended
Diagnostic Subtypes	Combined and partial subtypes based on symptomatology Combined: 6 or more from the IN domain and 6 or more from the HI domain Inattentive: 6 or more from the IN domain and less than 6 from hyperactive/impulsive domain Hyperactive/ Impulsive: 6 or more from HI domain and less than 6 from the IN domain	Subtypes based on comorbid disorder diagnosis Disturbance of activity and attention (without conduct disorder) Hyperkinetic conduct disorder (with conduct disorder)

2.2 **Epidemiology**

The differences between countries in the prevalence of ADHD and HKD have generated considerable controversy. However, when operational definitions of ADHD/HKD are used, differences between countries are small. A recent systematic review on ADHD prevalence during childhood and adolescence based on 102 studies from across all world regions calculated an overall prevalence of ADHD of 5.3%. The prevalence for children was 6.5% and for adolescents 2.7% (Polanczyk et al., 2007). Differences between studies were mainly accounted for by:

- the use of differing diagnostic criteria (DSM-III, DSM-III-R, DSM-IV, or ICD-10)
- the source of information and the method used to gather diagnostic information (best-estimate procedure, parents, 'and rule', 'or rule', teachers, or subjects; behaviour checklist, structured interview, etc.)
- the requirement, or not, for impairment to be present in order for the diagnosis to be made.

. After adjustments are made to account for these methodological issues, the estimates from North America and Europe are not significantly different from each other.

The prevalence of the more restrictive ICD-10 hyperkinetic disorder diagnosis has been estimated to be around 1.5% in school-age children. In clinical practice, the rate of recognition of a disorder, the administrative prevalence, often differs from the epidemiological prevalence. Administrative prevalence depends on factors that affect referral and access to service and cultural factors that influence tolerance of the symptoms, as well as on the actual presence of symptoms.

Estimates of the prevalence of adult ADHD vary significantly. A population survey conducted in the United States estimated a prevalence of adult ADHD of 4.4% (Kessler et al., 2006), which is comparable with a large cross-national survey by Fayyad et al. (2007), which documented a prevalence of DSM-IV adult ADHD of around 3.4% (range 1.2–7.3%) across ten countries in the Americas, Europe, and the Middle East.

The impact of ethnic and socio-economic issues on the prevalence rates of ADHD has been much less well investigated. However, in general it appears that ADHD is a worldwide disorder and that, as long as similar methodologies are used, the prevalence rates are similar in most ethnic communities (Coghill et al., 2008).

2.3 **Clinical presentation**

Clinical presentation of ADHD is highly variable. Some patients have only very minor symptoms, while others may have severe impairments. Diagnosis requires that there should be clear evidence of clinically significant impairment in social, academic, or occupational functioning. Impairment implies not only a higher severity or frequency of symptoms but also interference with functioning in the major life domains of the child, e. g. at home, at school, with friends, or elsewhere.

The predominantly inattentive type is relatively more common in females and, together with the combined type, seems to have a higher impact on academic performance. Children with the predominantly hyperactive-impulsive type are more aggressive and impulsive than those with the predominantly inattentive type of ADHD, and tend to be unpopular and highly rejected by their peers. The combined type causes more impairment to global functioning, comparatively to the other two types.

Clinical presentation may also vary according to age and stage of development (see below). In addition, there are cultural differences in the level of activity and inattention that are regarded as a problem (Taylor *et al.*, 2004).

2.4 **Differential diagnoses**

It is important to note that ADHD/HKD symptoms are not specific to the disorder (see Box 2.2). As isolated symptoms inattention, hyperactivity, and impulsivity may be the final path for many problems related to conflicts with parents and/or peers, inappropriate educational systems, or may even be associated with other disorders that are commonly observed in childhood and adolescence. Therefore, a careful assessment of each symptom in the child's history and consideration of a range of differential diagnoses and co-existing conditions are always necessary for the diagnosis of ADHD (see Chapter 4, sections 4.2.1, 4.2.2). For instance, a child may show difficulty following instructions due to an oppositional defiant behaviour towards parents or teachers, which characterizes a symptom of an oppositional defiant dis-order instead of ADHD. In most cases differential diagnoses can be addressed by a careful initial assessment, however, in some situations observation over time is required (Taylor *et al.*, 2004).

Box 2.2 Potential differential (or comorbid) diagnoses

- Oppositional defiant disorder or conduct disorders (may sometimes give difficulties in the differential diagnosis)
- Pervasive developmental disorders
- Anxiety and mood disorders
- Acute adjustment disorders
- Attachment disorders
- Learning disorders (differential diagnosis to inattention)
- Mental retardation (does not exclude the diagnosis of ADHD)
- Family conflict, bullying, or child abuse can also present with ADHD-like symptoms (alternative explanations or co-occurring problems)
- Chromosomal, metabolic, neurologica, or somatic disorders (e.g., fragile X syndrome; 22q11 deletion syndrome, petit mal epilepsy, migraine, hyperthyreosis) can masquerade as ADHD
- Medication, especially anticonvulsants, antihistamines, sympatho-mimetics, steroids.

2.5 **Comorbid disorders**

The co-existence of several other types of psychopathology along with ADHD is very common in clinical and community samples (up to 80% in clinical samples) (Biederman & Faraone, 2005). Thus, clinicians should be prepared to encounter a wide range of psychiatric symptoms in the course of managing patients with ADHD.

In Figure 2.1, the ADHD comorbid profiles in three different clinical samples from Brazil (Souza et al., 2004), the US (MTA Cooperative Group, 1999), and Europe (Steinhausen et al., 2006) are depicted suggesting a worldwide consistent profile of high comorbidity in ADHD samples.

2.5.1 **Oppositional defiant disorder and conduct disorder**

Both clinical and epidemiological studies show a high prevalence of comorbidity between ADHD and disruptive behavioural disorders (conduct disorder and oppositional defiant disorder), which ranges from 30 to 80% (median odds ratio of 10). Conduct disorder and oppositional defiant disorder should often be seen, not necessarily as a differential diagnosis or a comorbid condition, but as a complication. Hyperactive behaviour is a high risk factor for developing conduct disorder, even in children who showed a pure pattern of hyperactivity without conduct disorder at the beginning of their problems. Conduct disorder does not give rise to ADHD in the same way (Angold et al., 1999; Biederman & Faraone, 2005).

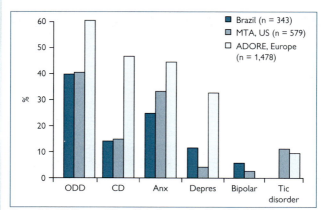

Figure 2.1 ADHD comorbid profile in three studies: The MTA (MTA Cooperative Group, 1999), the ADORE (Steinhausen et al., 2006), and Souza et al. (2004; Brazil). Data are presented as percentages. In the Brazilian study, the comorbid profile is described only for one site (Porto Alegre) and no information is reported for tic disorders. In the MTA, only ADHD-combined type is included and several restrictions were applied to enroll patients with severe mood disorders. No information is available for bipolar disorder in the ADORE study. ODD=Oppositional defiant disorder; CD=conduct disorder; Anx=anxiety; Depres=depression. Reproduced from Coghill et al. (2008), with kind permission from Karger, Basel.

2.5.2 **Emotional disorders**

There is also a significant comorbidity with anxiety disorders (up to 25%; median odds ratio of 3.0) and depression (15–20%; median odds ratio of 5.5). The reasons for the frequent coexistence of hyperactivity and problems of anxiety and depression are not well understood. Some children may develop low self esteem and insecurity as a result of failures at school and interpersonal relationships. Emotional disorders are often overlooked (Angold et al., 1999; Biederman & Faraone, 2005).

2.5.3 **Bipolar disorder**

Many children with ADHD have extreme and uncontrolled mood changes and a specialist referral is advised because the problems are often complex. Comorbidity with bipolar disorder needs to be considered, but the relationship between ADHD and paediatric bipolar disorder remains controversial (the two main areas of controversy are the role of cardinal symptoms—grandiosity and euphoria versus irritability and the relevance of episodicity for the diagnosis). Current evidence suggests that severe, non-episodic irritability may rather be a variant of depression and children and adolescents with severe, non-episodic irritability seem to differ from those with bipolar disorder in longitudinal course, family history, and pathophysiological mechanisms. Thus, it is recommended that the diagnoses of bipolar disorder or bipolar disorder not otherwise specified should only be made in the presence of identifiable manic or hypomanic episodes, including a distinct change from baseline mood with concurrent alterations in behaviour (Baroni et al., 2009).

2.5.4 **Pervasive developmental disorders**

While ICD-10 and DSM-IV preclude the diagnosis of ADHD, if problems are better explained by autism or other pervasive developmental disorders, ADHD and symptoms of autistic spectrum disorders can often co-exist. Several studies have shown social deficits, peer relationship and empathy problems to be common in ADHD. Clinically, children with ADHD and autistic symptoms may respond to stimulants (though caution is needed in view of possible adverse effects). It is therefore desirable to recognize both types of symptoms when they are present (Taylor et al., 2004).

2.5.5 **Tic disorders**

Children with ADHD have an increased risk to develop comorbid tic disorders during their early school years. Similarly, about half of the cases with chronic tics or Tourette syndrome also meet criteria for ADHD (Freeman et al., 2006). In these cases, the degree of psychosocial impairment is usually determined by ADHD. Usually, ADHD starts about 2 to 3 years before the tics, while in a smaller proportion of cases ADHD can be seen only after tic onset.

2.5.6 **Substance abuse**

Several studies have found evidence for earlier and increased use of alcohol, tobacco, and substance abuse in adolescents with ADHD compared to controls; a high prevalence of drug abuse or dependency is reported in adulthood (9–40%). Whilst controlling for comorbid disorders (particularly conduct disorder) substantially weakens this association, there is some evidence that non-comorbid ADHD in adolescents and adults does act as an independent risk factor for substance use disorders (Szobot et al., 2007).

2.5.7 **Language delays, learning disorders, and neuropsychological deficits**

In addition, children with ADHD may experience a wide range of other problems. Population studies suggest that mental retardation may be more common (up to 5–10 times) in ADHD than in children without ADHD (Simonoff et al., 2007).

Patients with ADHD are at risk for co-existing language disorders. Some studies have suggested that girls with ADHD may be particularly at risk of language delay and current co-existing language disorders.

A variety of learning problems are associated with ADHD that need to be addressed separately both as regards assessment and interventions. About 25–40% of all patients with ADHD have major reading and writing difficulties. The overlap of ADHD and reading disorders seems to be largely accounted for by genetic overlap. Similarly, there is a considerable overlap between ADHD and mathematics disorder.

Furthermore, ADHD is associated with weaknesses in multiple neuropsychological domains, i.e., global intellectual functioning, executive functions (motor response inhibition, working memory, vigilance, and planning), processing speed, response variability, and a motivational style that is characterized by a significant aversion to delay (see also section 3.2.2.2), even when comorbid disorders are excluded or controlled. Executive function weaknesses are associated with inattention symptoms more specifically and may be more severe in those individuals with ADHD and comorbid reading disorder. However, individual differences in executive functions do not explain a high amount of variance in ADHD symptoms (Willcutt et al., 2008).

2.5.8 **Developmental coordination disorder**

ADHD is often accompanied by problems in sensory motor coordination, especially seen as poor handwriting, clumsiness, poor performance in sports, and marked delays in achieving motor milestones. Many children with ADHD fulfill criteria of a developmental coordination disorder. Interestingly, the rate is equally high in those with severe and moderate variants of ADHD, and also in those with subclinical variants of the disorder (Reiersen et al., 2008).

2.5.9 **Sleep problems**

Children with ADHD are more likely to have sleep problems. These problems include difficulties in falling asleep and more disruptions during the course of the night (Cortese et al., 2006).

Treatment considerations of several specific groups are described in chapters 5 and 6.

2.6 **Gender aspects**

ADHD is more common in boys than in girls. In the systematic review mentioned above including 102 epidemiological studies, the pooled ADHD prevalence for boys was 2.45 times higher than that detected for girls. In clinic-referred samples, ratios between 6:1 and 9:1 might be found but this may decrease with age.

The increased prevalence among girls found in epidemiological samples compared to clinical samples, suggests that there may be greater barriers to recognition, referral and diagnosis of ADHD in girls than in boys or that the clinical severity may differ between both genders (Gaub & Carlson, 1997).

The latter explanation seems more likely; among children with ADHD identified from epidemiological samples, girls with ADHD appear to be less impaired in a number of domains, such as hyperactivity, inattention, impulsivity, and externalizing problems than non-referred boys with ADHD; however, girls and boys with ADHD identified from clinic-referred samples are more similar than different, except for a trend for greater severity of inattention, greater intellectual impairments, and more internalizing problems among girls. Thus, they are more often diagnosed as predominantly inattentive than boys with ADHD. Developmental patterns may differ. With age, girls with ADHD seem to be increasingly rejected by peers while the social status of boys with ADHD remains stable (Gaub & Carlson *et al.*, 1997).

2.7 **Prognosis, course and outcome**

Children and adolescents with ADHD may face problems in many different domains, including school problems and academic under-achievement, low self-esteem, difficulties in parent-child interactions, sibling interactions and peer relationships, and poorer psychosocial adjustment. Furthermore, they are at increased risk for all types of accidents from early childhood. Social difficulties may be more extensive if the child also has ODD or CD. However, ADHD as such is a strong risk factor for later psychiatric diagnosis, antisocial behaviour, and social and peer problems, even after allowing for a co-existent conduct disorder.

Outcomes over the lifespan differ widely. Changes in symptoms across childhood and adolescence may be a consequence of natural developmental processes seen in all children, but symptoms may also diminish due to learned skills, coping strategies, and environmental restructuring.

2.7.1 **Preschoolers**

Although ADHD is most frequently identified during elementary school years, epidemiologic data suggest that core symptoms are frequently present from early childhood and may be noticed as early as 3 years of age. Difficult early temperament features may even be precursors. Of the core symptoms, hyperactivity is likely more noticeable than symptoms of inattention which may not become apparent until the child enters elementary school. While current data suggest that once age-adjustments have been made, there is some equivalence between preschool and school-based ADHD in terms of symptom structure and impairment (Döpfner *et al.*, 2004), the diagnosis of ADHD should be made with caution before the age of 6 years, because more intense activity and a short attention span may occur more frequently in normal preschool children than in school-aged children and the developmental course and its persistence may still be more variable.

2.7.2 **Adults**

While ADHD symptoms, as a whole, decline with age and hyperactivity-impulsivity symptoms tend to diminish after puberty or present differently with age, symptoms of inattention do not, and symptoms of other disorders, such as conduct and anxiety disorders, increase with age (Faraone et al., 2006). A very large majority (60-85%) of children with ADHD will continue to meet criteria for the disorder during the teenage years. Longitudinal studies have documented that ADHD/HKD persists through childhood into adolescence and adulthood in many cases. The extent to which ADHD persists into adulthood depends heavily on how it is defined. About 65% of children with ADHD experience partial remission in adulthood (with significant clinical impairments), and the full ADHD diagnosis is met in approximately 15% at age 25, when full diagnostic criteria were required (Faraone et al., 2006).

The risk factors determining the persistence of ADHD diagnosis in adults remain unclear. However, some studies suggested that higher persistence is associated with:

- family history of ADHD
- adversities during childhood, including family adversity
- increased severity of ADHD symptoms
- presence of comorbidities.

Evidence from population studies points to substantially elevated rates of comorbid psychiatric disorders in adults with ADHD (Kessler et al., 2006). Adults with ADHD have a particularly high risk for antisocial personality disorder (up to 10 times that of controls, i.e. about 20% of the cases) and comorbid substance abuse disorder (4–8 times that of controls). Compared to control populations, adults with ADHD have also elevated rates of mood disorder (2–6 times), anxiety disorders (2–4 times), relationship dysfunction (2 times) and learning disorder. Additional psychopathology may include disorganized behaviour related to executive function deficits in attention, behavioural inhibition, verbal long-term memory, problem-solving ability and planning and emotional dysregulation is common in adulthood (Hervey et al., 2004).

While many children with ADHD will grow up without persistent problems, patients with ADHD are at increased risk of a worse outcome across the life span (Kessler et al., 2006). Thus, adult ADHD is associated with:

- higher rates of several psychiatric comorbidities, such as disruptive behaviour disorders, anxiety, mood disorders, and substance use disorders
- low self-concept and low self-esteem

- significant deficits in work performance and greater levels of unemployment, sub-employment, and job changes compared to control groups. Workplace safety is also an issue, with ADHD associated with increased risk of workplace accidents and injuries
- family dysfunction such as divorce and poor quality of family relations; difficulties in peer relationship and family functioning that often affect children and adolescents with ADHD frequently extend into adulthood. Thus, adults with ADHD also report higher rates of separation and divorce. Parents with ADHD may face problems in parenting effectively due to their symptomatology
- accidents and driving impairments; adults with ADHD are at greater risk of adverse driving outcomes such as greater numbers of motor vehicle accidents and traffic violations
- increased sexual risk-taking behaviours; adolescents and adults with ADHD may take greater sexual risks, e.g., more teen pregnancies
- social and legal problems; although the vast majority of individuals with ADHD will never become involved with crime, research indicates a consistent association between ADHD and delinquency, antisocial and criminal behaviour, and recidivism; it appears that the symptoms of hyperactivity-impulsivity, but not inattention, contribute to the risk for criminal involvement over and above the risk associated with early conduct problems alone.

- Overall, burdens for families as well as the economic costs for society caused by ADHD are substantial.

References

American Psychiatric Association (2000). Diagnostic and statistical manual of mental disorders, fourth edition, revised (DSM-IV-TR) Washington DC: American Psychiatric Association.

American Psychiatric Association (1994). Diagnostic and Statistical Manual of Mental Disorders. Washington, American Psychiatric Association.

Angold A, Costello EJ, Erkanli A, (1999). Comorbidity. *Journal of Child Psychology & Psychiatry & Allied Disciplines* **40**(1): 57–87.

Baroni A, Lunsford JR, Luckenbaugh DA, Towbin KE, Leibenluft E (2009). Practitioner Review: The assessment of bipolar disorder in children and adolescents. *Journal of Child Psychology and Psychiatry*. doi:10.1111/j.1469–7610.2008.01953.x.

Biederman J, Faraone SV, (2005). Attention-deficit hyperactivity disorder. *Lancet* **366**(9481): 237–48.

Coghill D, Rohde LA, Banaschewski T (2008): Attention-Deficit/Hyperactivity Disorder. Banaschewski T, Rohde LA (eds): *Biological Child Psychiatry. Recent Trends and Developments. Adv Biol Psychiatry.* Basel, Karger, vol 24, pp. 1–20.

Cortese S, Konofal E, Yateman N, Mouren MC, Lecendreux M (2006). Sleep and alertness in children with attention-deficit/hyperactivity disorder: a systematic review of the literature. *Sleep* **29**(4): 504–11.

Döpfner M, Rothenberger A, Sonuga-Barke E. (2004). Areas for future investment in the field of ADHD: preschoolers and clinical networks. *Eur Child Adolesc Psychiatry* **13** Suppl 1: I130–5.

Faraone SV, Biederman J, Mick E (2006). The age-dependent decline of attention deficit hyperactivity disorder: a meta-analysis of follow-up studies. *Psychological Medicine* **36**(2):159–65.

Fayyad J, De Graaf R, Kessler R, Alonso J, Angermeyer M, Demyttenaere K, De Girolamo G, Haro JM, Karam EG, Lara C, Lepine JP, Ormel J, Posada-Villa J, Zaslavsky AM, Jin R (2007). Cross-national prevalence and correlates of adult attention-deficit hyperactivity disorder. *Br J Psychiatry* **190**(5):402–9.

Freeman R, Consortium TSID, (2007). Tic disorders and ADHD: answers from a world-wide clinical dataset on Tourette syndrome *European Child and Adolescent Psychiatry* 2007 **16** Supp 9:I/15-I/23

Gaub M, Carlson C L (1997). Gender differences in ADHD: a meta-analysis and critical review. *J Am Acad Child Adolesc Psychiatry* **36**(8): 1036–45.

Hervey AS, Epstein JN, Curry JF (2004). Neuropsychology of adults with attention-deficit/hyperactivity disorder: a meta-analytic review. *Neuropsychology* **18**(3): 485–503.

Kessler RC, Adler L, Barkley R, Biederman J, Conners CK, Demler O, Faraone SV, Greenhill LL, Howes MJ, Secnik K, Spencer T, Ustun TB, Walters EE, Zaslavsky AM (2006). The prevalence and correlates of adult ADHD in the United States: results from the National Comorbidity Survey Replication. *Am J Psychiatry* **163**(4):716–23.

MTA Cooperative Group (1999): A 14-month randomized clinical trial of treatment strategies for attentiondeficit/ hyperactivity disorder. Multimodal Treatment Study of Children with ADHD. *Arch Gen Psychiatry* **56**: 1073–1086.

Polanczyk G, Lima MS, Horta BL, Biederman J, Rohde LA (2007): The worldwide prevalence of attention deficit/hyperactivity disorder: a systematic review and meta-regression analyses. *Am J Psychiatry* **164**: 942–8.

Reiersen AM, Constantino JN, Todd RD (2008). Co-occurrence of motor problems and autistic symptoms in attention-deficit/hyperactivity disorder. *J Am Acad Child Adolesc Psychiatry* **47**(6): 662–72.

Schachar R., Chen S, Crosbie J, Goos L, Ickowicz A, Charach A (2007). Comparison of the predictive validity of hyperkinetic disorder and attention deficit hyperactivity disorder. *J Can Acad Child Adolesc Psychiatry* **16**(2): 90–100.

Simonoff E, Pickles A, Wood N, Gringras P, Chadwick O (2007). ADHD symptoms in children with mild intellectual disability. *J Am Acad Child Adolesc Psychiatry* **46**(5): 591–600.

Souza I, Pinheiro MA, Denardin D, Mattos P, Rohde LA (2004): Attention-deficit/hyperactivity disorder and comorbidity in Brazil: comparison between two referred samples. *Eur Child Adolesc Psychiatry* **13**: 243–8.

Steinhausen HC, Novik TS, Baldursson G, Curatolo P, Lorenzo MJ, Rodrigues Pereira R, Ralston SJ, Rothenberger A; ADORE Study Group (2006): Co-existing psychiatric problems in ADHD in the ADORE cohort. *Eur Child Adolesc Psychiatry* **15** Suppl 1: i25–i29.

Swanson JM, Sergeant JA, Taylor E, Sonuga-Barke EJS, Jensen PJ, Cantwell DP (1998). Attention-deficit hyperactivity disorder and hyperkinetic disorder. *Lancet* **351**: 9100:429–33.

Szobot CM, Rohde LA, Bukstein O, Molina BS, Martins C, Ruaro P, Pechansky F (2007): Is attention-deficit/hyperactivity disorder associated with illicit substance use disorders in male adolescents? A community-based case-control study. *Addiction* **102**(7): 1122–30.

Taylor E. Döpfner, M, Sergeant J, Asherson P, Banaschewski T, Buitelaar J, Coghill D, Danckaerts M, Rothenberger A, Sonuga-Barke E, Steinhausen HC, Zuddas A (2004). European clinical guidelines for hyperkinetic disorder—first upgrade. *Eur Child Adolesc Psychiatry* **13** Suppl 1: I7–30.

Willcutt EG, Sonuga-Barke EJS, Nigg JT, Sergeant JA (2008): Recent Developments in Neuropsychological Models of Childhood Psychiatric Disorders. Banaschewski T, Rohde LA (eds): Biological Child Psychiatry. Recent Trends and Developments. *Adv Biol Psychiatry*. Basel, Karger, vol 24, pp. 195–226.

World Health Organization (1992). *International Classification of Diseases* (ICD-10) 10th Edition. Geneva.

Chapter 3

Pathogenesis

Edmund Sonuga-Barke

Key points

- ADHD appears to have a complex etiology. There are multiple genetic and environmental risk factors of small effect that act in concert to create a spectrum of neurobiological liability.
- Understanding the etiology of ADHD will depend crucially on modelling the interplay between genetic and environmental risk factors in terms of both gene-environment correlations and interactions.
- Cognitive impairment in ADHD is not fixed but appears to be highly context dependent suggesting that an individual's state and levels of motivation in relation to a task or setting are important in determining performance.
- ADHD is not a single pathophysiological entity and there may be different subgroups of individual patients with different profiles of neuropsychological impairment.

ADHD has a complex pathogenesis. A growing body of evidence is supportive of a model in which multiple genetic and environmental factors interact during early development to create a neuro-biological liability to disorder, the expression of which is mediated by alterations within different and diverse neural networks and deficits in the neuropsychological functions which these subserve. Furthermore, it is becoming increasingly clear that there are likely to be marked individual differences within the ADHD population in the extent to which particular genetic, environmental, and neuro-pathophysiological processes are implicated. The possibility that the pathways between risk and disorder can be moderated by environmental factors is also being taken increasingly seriously. Furthermore, the timing of exposure to environmental factors needs to be considered.

3.1 **Etiology**

3.1.1 **Genetics**

Genetic factors are implicated in ADHD—although the mechanisms of action are not understood at present, they are without doubt complicated: ADHD is not a genetic disorder in any simple sense. ADHD is familial and highly heritable. Twin studies suggesting heritability estimates of 60 to 90% (Thapar et al., 2000) raised initial expectations that it would be relatively easy to identify the gene or patterns of genes responsible for the condition. This has not been the case. Candidate gene studies focusing in particular on genes regulating neurotransmitter systems thought to be implicated in ADHD have identified a number of replicable associations with dopamine genes with putative functional significance for ADHD (D4 and D5 receptors and the Dopamine Transporter; Faraone et al., 2005) with suggestive but largely un-replicated evidence for a role of genes in other neurotransmitter systems (e.g., norepinephrine and serotonin systems). However, these effects are extremely small, accounting even when aggregated for a small fraction of variation in ADHD within the population. This picture is reinforced by non-hypothesis driven quantitative searches for genes. Different linkage studies have been largely unsuccessful in identifying common disease susceptibility loci for ADHD (e.g., Hebebrand et al., 2006). Genome wide association scans, including many hundred's of thousands of genetic markers, while identifying new candidates worthy of further study, have so far failed to find good evidence for effects significant at the level of the whole genome (Lasky-Su et al., 2008). See Box 3.1.

The mismatch between the high heritability of ADHD revealed by twin studies and the general lack of evidence for genetic main effects from molecular genetic studies is open to a number of interpretations. First, it seems unlikely that there are any major ADHD genes accounting on their own for a substantial proportion (e.g., >5%) of ADHD variation in the population. Second, many genes of very small effect are likely to be implicated in ADHD, individually and in combination with each other. Third, that environmental factors may play a more important role in the etiology of ADHD than previously thought and that genetic environmental risks likely interact in creating the risk for ADHD. Initial studies, reviewed below, of the interaction between specific risk alleles and individual putative environmental risk factors provide initial evidence to support this view. Finally, that etiological heterogeneity is high in ADHD with individual patients being affected by different combinations of genetic and risk factors in different ways. This means that although the effect of a gene when judged across the whole ADHD population may be

> **Box 3.1 The genetic basis of ADHD**
>
> - ADHD is highly familial and heritable
> - Replicated candidate genes are primarily linked to the dopamine system (e.g. DRD4 and DAT1)
> - Effects of individual genes are small—ADHD is genetically heterogeneous and has a complex genetic architecture
> - Genome-wide approaches have not been sufficiently powered to identify novel genes.

small and of limited importance, it may be extremely important for a sub-group of patients. Therefore a major challenge for future ADHD research involves attempts to partition this heterogeneity to produce more etiologically homogeneous groupings in which the role of specific genes and environments may be more powerful. This could be achieved be exploring gene x environmental effects (as described above and reviewed below) as genes may only be implicated in individuals exposed to a specific environment (and vice versa). It could also be achieved by using alternative phenotypes within the broader ADHD category that might define a more etiologically homogeneous subtype. This can be done at the clinical or (exo-)phenotypic level where the genetic factors implicated in patients with different clinical profiles (more severe vs less severe or inattentive vs hyperactive impulsive) can be investigated. It can also be done at the endo-phenotypic level where the genetic profile of patients with different neuro-biological or -psychological characteristics can be explored (Doyle et al., 2005).

3.1.2 **Environment**
The strategy of studying genes in isolation from environments was never likely to be optimal in the case of a complex and heterogeneous disorder such as ADHD. Indeed evidence from many different sources now supports an important role for pre-, peri- and post-natal environmental factors in the pathogenesis of ADHD (Taylor & Rogers, 2005). See Box 3.2.

3.1.2.1 *Pre-natal factors*
Pre-natal factors associated with maternal lifestyle during pregnancy, have been implicated in ADHD etiology. The association with maternal smoking during pregnancy has been replicated in a number of studies. Maternal alcohol consumption may also be important but these effects are less marked if foetal alcohol syndrome is accounted for (Linnet et al., 2003). The effects of pre-natal exposure to both prescribed therapeutic and non-prescribed drugs of abuse (i.e., cocaine) have been investigated, although evidence is inconclusive and their effects hard to disentangle from maternal mental state during pregnancy.

Evidence that maternal mental health might be important also comes from replicated finding that maternal stress during pregnancy may play a role, possibly via its effects on cortisol secretion (O'Connor *et al.*, 2003). Peri-natal factors have also been implicated with a two fold increase in ADHD in very low birth weight children and an increased rate of pregnancy and birth complications in ADHD individuals (Taylor & Rogers, 2005).

The situation with regard to the role of environmental factors is in some ways similar to that found for genetics: There are multiple pre- and peri-natal environmental influences of small effect implicated in the pathogenesis of the ADHD. Teasing apart the influence of individual risks for ADHD is extremely challenging because of the inevitable inter-relations between individual environmental risks and other risks relating to lifestyle, social class/economic adversity and maternal personality. Furthermore, this mix of adversity and risk is also likely to be correlated with genetic risk and it may be that the reported effects are simply the product of correlations between environments and genes and the patterns of environmental adversity are marking an increase in genetic risk. However, even in designs that allow genetic factors to be controlled environmental main effects persist. The mechanisms by which these pre- and peri-natal factors operate during the pathogenesis of ADHD are currently unknown.

3.1.2.2 *The post-natal environment*

Factors within the postnatal environment also play a role. The child's physical environment seems important. For instance, diet may play a small but significant role. Recent RCTs support the idea that these are general effect that extends beyond the clinically diagnosed and those who seem to be influenced by idiosyncratic allergic reactions (McCann *et al.*, 2007). A role for malnutrition and dietary deficiency in ADHD has been proposed. Variation in fatty acids intake has been suggested but requires systematic study. Iron exposure has been implicated in individual cases.

Although often overlooked in models of ADHD pathogenesis, the postnatal social environment may play an important role. In extremis this may take the form of a primary cause as appears to be the case for some children exposed to extremely depriving institutional environments during their early formative years. In the English and Romanian Adoptees study children who spent their early years in Romanian institutions had significantly increased rates of ADHD including pervasive and persistent overactivity and inattention (Rutter *et al.*, 2007). More generally, the social, and more specifically the family environment, appears to be implicated in the course and persistence of the condition rather than its onset. ADHD is associated with negative, intrusive and harsh parenting but typically these are viewed as a response to the child's challenging behaviour rather than a cause of the disorder. However, the relationship is likely to be complex and the possibility that inappropriate parenting can exacerbate the ADHD presentation, especially with regard to the emergence of significant impairment, should not be ruled out (Seipp & Johnston, 2005). However, it seems clear that inappropriate parenting is associated with the onset of comorbidity (Ostrander & Herman, 2006) in ADHD children. There is currently little data on the power of 'good' parenting to alter ADHD trajectories. However, a supportive family environment may help with the development of coping strategies that reduce functional impairment and improve quality of life. Data from randomized controlled trials of parenting provide support for the idea that positively therapeutic environments can lead to clinically significant remission of both core ADHD symptoms and reductions in oppositional defiant behaviour (Sonuga-Barke et al., 2001). Furthermore, controlled exposure to cognitive training may improve functioning in core deficits which in turn reduces ADHD symptoms (Klingberg et al., 2005).

3.1.3 Gene-environment interplay

Given the limited explanatory power of simple main effects of genetic and environmental risks, more complex models of the etiology of ADHD incorporating gene-environment interplay need to be considered. In this regard there are a number of important considerations. First, there is almost certainly gene-environment correlation in ADHD. This might take two forms, examples of which have been mentioned above. First, risk environments experienced by the child may be correlated with genes shared with parents as in the case where maternal smoking during pregnancy may be correlated with genetic risk for ADHD shared by parent and child (passive gene-environment correlation). Second, risk environments may be evoked

---

Box 3.2 The environmental basis of ADHD

- The environment is also important in ADHD
- Prenatal exposures to adverse fetal environments and negative perinatal experiences increase the risk of ADHD by a significant degree
- The evidence for a moderate effect of maternal smoking during pregnancy is strong while the effects of alcohol exposure and maternal stress are less clear cut but are potentially important
- Post-natal diet may be more important than once thought
- The social environment within the family may play an important role in developmental complications such as the development of oppositional defiant disorder.

by genetically based characteristics in the child as when ADHD symptoms elicit maternal hostility (active gene-environment correlations). Little evidence to support this view exists but despite this many assume that these gene-environment correlations make an important contribution to explaining ADHD.

Emerging evidence does support gene x environment interactions in ADHD (Thapar *et al.*, 2007). In gene x environment interactions the effect of a gene is moderated by exposure to a particular environmental risk (or vice versa) so that its effects are larger following risk exposure than where no exposure occurs. Most studies so far have focused on the dopamine genes, DAT1 and DRD4, providing evidence that exposure to pre-natal risks such as in-utero exposure to smoking and alcohol during pregnancy moderates the effect of these genes (e.g., Becker *et al.*, 2008). Serotonin genes (e.g., 5-HTT-LPR) interact with social adversity to increase risk for externalizing problems including (Retz *et al.*, 2008) ADHD. How might these effects operate? There are a number of hypotheses. First, environmental exposures may moderate gene expression—i.e., 'switch on' or 'switch off' a particular ADHD susceptibility gene. Alternatively, a gene may alter the degree of exposure to an environment, the way it is experienced or increase resilience to its negative effects. Understanding epigenetic mechanisms in ADHD represents an important research priority.

Our current knowledge of ADHD etiology provides some pointers for clinicians to help them to advise patients and their parents on the cases of ADHD. Some of these are outlined in Table 3.1.

3.2 **Pathophysiology**

3.2.1 **Brain structure**

Recent meta-analyses of MRI structural findings support alterations in a broad range of brain regions of ADHD patients. ADHD children have significantly smaller brains in general, with the largest reduction in specific structures being found for cerebellum, corpus callosum, cerebrum (especially the right lobe), right caudate and specific frontal regions (Valera *et al.*, 2007). Grey matter differences have also been shown in the putamen/globus pallidus (Ellison-Wright *et al.*, 2008). There is also evidence of cortical thinning in the region of the dorso-lateral prefrontal cortex. Studies of white matter integrity using diffusion tensor imaging have found abnormalities in the frontal and cerebellar fiber pathways thought to sub-serve cognitive functions implicated in ADHD (Makris *et al.*, 2007). The impact of medication on brain structure has not been studied sufficiently systematically to properly tease out disease related and treatment related effects.

Table 3.1 Clinical implications of current understanding of the etiology of ADHD

Environmental influences to include in the clinical history:

Pregnancy:
- alcohol
- smoking
- prescribed drugs (esp. psychotropics and anticonvulsants)
- illegal drugs
- toxaemia, haemorrhage
- rashes and fever
- psychological stress
- fetal distress

Perinatal:
- gestational age and birth weight
- Apgar below 5
- hypoglycaemia
- respiratory distress
- encephalopathy (e.g. fits)

Postnatal
- neurological illness or injury
- severe deprivation

Genetic counseling:

When counseling is requested, always:
- Clarify what parents wish to know
- Ask about affected relatives (and if there are many test as for low IQ below)
- Physical examination for specific genetic disorders

In the presence of ordinary IQ:
- No case for molecular genetic screening
- Recurrence risk substantially raised for siblings
- Exact prediction not possible

In the presence of intellectual disability:
- Routine chromosome examination
- Fragile-X
- Other specific tests (e.g. 22q11) if condition suspected clinically
- Consider FISH* for telomeric rearrangements

* FISH: fluorescence in-situ hybridization

Table provided by E.Taylor

3.2.2 Neurochemistry

Genetic, imaging and pharmacological studies implicate catecholamine (especially dopamine) dysregulation in ADHD (Oades *et al.*, 2005). SPECT and PET are consistent with the notion of dopamine and norepinephrine depletion in ADHD (Spencer *et al.*, 2005) a view consistent with the evidence that dopamine (DA) and norepinephrine (NE) agonists (e.g., methylphenidate and atomoxetine) reduce ADHD symptoms by increasing extracellular DA and NE. Brain networks implicated

Box 3.3 The Neurobiology of ADHD

- Structural imaging studies show that ADHD children's brains are significantly smaller than unaffected controls
- The pre-frontal cortex, basal ganglia and cerebellum are differentially affected–although effects are modest
- Evidence for reduced connectivity in white matter tracts in key brain areas is emerging
- Functional imaging studies identify a wide range of abnormalities in brain activity during task performance
- Effects are task specific with effects most consistent in the pre-frontal cortex and the neo-striatum on tests of inhibitory control
- Alternations within ventral networks (orbito-frontal cortex— ventral stratum) have been observed on reward processing tasks
- Genetic, pharmacological, imaging, and animal models highlight the key role of dopamine dysregulation in the neurobiological basis of ADHD.

implicated in ADHD deficits are heavily innervated by DA and NE branches and medication improves functioning across neuropsychological domains deficient in ADHD (Boonstra et al., 2005) and normalize patterns of brain activity in key regions (e.g., Bush et al., 2008). The catecholamine hypothesis is also consonant with data implicating polymorphisms in genes affecting catecholamine function, especially dopamine. Furthermore, ADHD can be mimicked in animal models with pharmacological lesions and gene knockout of catecholamine systems (Madras et al., 2005). However, in interpreting this evidence one needs to be aware that catecholaminergic drugs can have effects in the absence of ADHD and that neural systems are complex and plastic: An altered neuro-chemical responses could be directly linked to causes of ADHD or could be a consequence of the condition or a marker of some more fundamental neuro-biologic process. Finally, it is extremely difficult to isolate the role of any one neuro-transmitter given the complex patterns of interaction between DA and NE and other systems such as serotonin and acetylcholine.

3.2.2 Brain function and neuropsychology

Data on brain structure and neurochemistry is consistent with the notion that alterations in multiple brain networks are implicated in ADHD and that one should therefore expect a degree of heterogeneity in patterns of brain dysfunction and neuropsychological impairment. It is becoming increasingly clear that this is the case.

3.2.2.1 *Executive dysfunction*

Consistent with the findings of structural alterations in fronto-striatal brain networks described above ADHD children are deficient in executive functions. At the neuropsychological level ADHD appears to be associated with deficits on a wide range of EF including those implicating inhibitory processes and interference control; but effects are also present for domains such as planning and working memory (Willcutt *et al.*, 2007). Functional imaging studies provide evidence of hypo-activation in the ventro- and dorso-lateral pre-frontal cortex and the neo-striatum (i.e., caudate and putamen; Rubia *et al.*, 1999). Positron Emission Tomography (PET) and SPECT report reduced glucose metabolism in frontal regions (Ernst *et al.*, 2003). Studies using event-related potentials (ERPs) and other electrophysiological paradigms provide further evidence for the executive dysfunction hypothesis (Fallgatter *et al.*, 2005). Interpreting these findings are complicated by the fact that (i) effect sizes are rarely larger than moderate and only a few ADHD children show a pervasive pattern of severe EF deficits; (ii) executive deficits are seen in children with other disorders; (iii) executive function tasks also involve more basic cognitive processes such as visual memory, timing, and basic attentional mechanisms such as orienting and alerting and deficits which are biologically plausible could therefore masquerade as executive deficits; (iv) executive function performance, given its effortful nature is highly sensitive to motivational and state related factors and these may be deficient in ADHD. The effect sizes for case-control differences across a range of neuropsychological constructs are shown in Figure 3.1 (Willcutt *et al.*, 2008).

3.2.2.2 *State dependent and dynamic nature of impairment in ADHD*

There is growing evidence that cognitive impairments in ADHD are not fixed and stable but vary from context to context and state to state. It has been proposed that this could be due to altered motivation in ADHD. It has been suggested that this is due to ADHD children being either under- and/or over-sensitive to contingencies (both positive and negative) and/or their manipulation or because they have difficulty making decisions about different outcomes (Luman *et al.*, 2005). The evidence for these explanations is currently not compelling. ADHD children do show an altered response to delayed reward manifest in their preference for immediacy over deled rewards, inappropriate response to the unexpected imposition of delay and/or extinction of reinforcement. They are biased towards task responses tied to immediate rewards; prefer reward immediacy to high reward rate or task ease. This has been explained in terms of altered

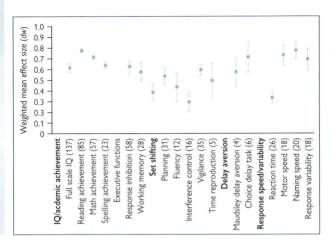

Figure 3.1 Weighted mean effect size of the difference between groups with and without ADHD (error bars indicate the 95% confidence interval for the weighted effect size). Numbers in parentheses indicate the number of studies that included the measure. Effect sizes were taken from previous meta-analyses and updated with results from studies published subsequent to the meta-analysis. The topics of the initial meta-anlaysis were IQ [13] academic achievement [161], overall executive functions [13, 20, 21], the stop-signal task [15], verbal and spatial working memory [17], Stroop interference control [14, 19], delay aversion [59], and processing speed [20]. Reproduced from Willcutt et al. (2008) with kind permission from Karger, Basel.

signalling of future rewards and/or perhaps an aversion to delay (Sonuga-Barke *et al.*, 2008). Consistent with these models imaging studies show hypoactivation in the ventral striatum during reward processing and hyperactivation in the amygdala when rewards are delayed (Plichta *et al.*, 2009).

The notion that ADHD children have state regulation deficits has also been developed out of the cognitive energetic model in which factors such as arousal, activation or effort are key modulators of cognitive performance. ADHD children are hypothesized to have particular difficulties in regulating their psycho-physiological state during periods of under- or over-activation. ADHD children may be less capable than controls at effectively allocating effort to regulate sub-optimal states (Sergeant, 2005). Key evidence in support of this claim comes from findings of the impact of event rate and support for the model comes from the repeated finding that ADHD performance deteriorates under low event rate conditions (van der Meere *et al.*, 2005).

3.2.2.3 *Are there pathophysiological subtypes?*

Given the heterogeneous nature of the pathogenesis of ADHD understanding the relationship between cognitive energetic, motivational and executive processes in ADHD is a major research goal (Sonuga-Barke *et al.*, 2008). It now seems highly unlikely that there is just one core deficit that explains the condition: that ADHD is a single patho-physiological entity. It's more likely that the disorder in different sub-grouping of the ADHD population is mediated by deficits in different and distinctive pathophysiological processes. Indeed deficits in executive and non-executive processes and motivational and energetic processes are relatively modest when seen at the level of diagnostic group as a whole and each type of deficit therefore may affect only a minority of cases. In one relevant study Solanto *et al.* (2001) found that that delay aversion and executive dysfunction were unrelated constructs each implicated in the disorder, but each affecting a different sub-section of ADHD individuals. The uncorrelated nature of executive dysfunction and delay aversion association has been found in other samples and has also been found in animal models. Following on from this a number of multiple pathway or process models have been proposed to account for this sort of data. The question of how other deficits associated with ADHD, such as timing and state regulation, map onto this dichotomy is currently unknown and needs to be investigated.

3.3 **In summary**

ADHD has a complex and heterogeneous pathogenesis. A reasonable working hypothesis is that multiple genes and environments interact to create a spectrum of biological risk the effects of which are mediated by a range of underlying neuro-biological deficits and moderated by significant environmental and genetic factors. The disorder is heterogeneous with different children displaying different psychopathological and pathophysiological profiles. While a developmental framework offers a way of understanding this complexity and partitioning this heterogeneity, the longitudinal data does not yet exist to disentangle to complex, dynamic and reciprocal patterns of interactions between factors and levels of analysis required. Figure 3.2 provides a illustration of a framework for understanding the complex pathogenesis of ADHD.

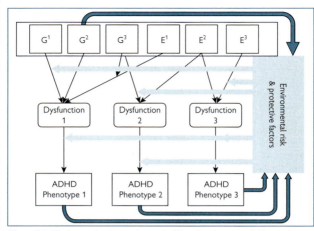

Figure 3.2 The interaction between genetic (G) and environmental (E) causal factors mediated by different forms of dysfunction in different patients leading to different clinical outcomes with reciprocal effects between causal factors, the social environment and the clinical outcome.

References

Becker K, El-Faddagh M, Schmidt MH, Esser G, Laucht M (2008). Interaction of dopamine transporter genotype with prenatal smoke exposure on ADHD symptoms. *J Ped* **152**: 263–9.

Boonstra AM, Kooij JSS, Oosterlaan J, Sergeant JA, Buitelaar JK (2005). Does methylphenidate improve inhibition and other cognitive abilities in adults with childhood-onset ADHD? *J Clin Exp Neuropsychol* **27**: 278–98.

Bush G, Spencer TJ, Holmes J, Shin LM, Valera EM, Seidman LJ, *et al.* (2008). Functional magnetic resonance imaging of methylphenidate and placebo in attention-deficit/hyperactivity disorder during the multi-source interference task. *Arch Gen Psychiatry* **65**: 102–14.

Doyle AE, Willcutt EG, Seidman, LJ, Biederman J, Chouinard VA, Silva J, *et al.* (2005). Attention-deficit/hyperactivity disorder endophenotypes. *Biol Psychiatry* **57**: 1324–35.

Ellison-Wright I, Ellison-Wright Z, Bullmore E (2008). Structural brain change in Attention Deficit Hyperactivity Disorder identified by meta-analysis. *BMC Psychiatry* **8**: 51.

Ernst M, Grant SJ, London ED, Contoreggi CS, Kimes AS, Spurgeaon L (2003). Decision making in adolescents with behaviour disorders and adults with substance abuse. *Am J Psychiatry* **160**: 33–40.

Fallgatter AJ, Ehlis AC, Rosler M, Strik WK, Blocher D, Herrmann MJ (2005). Diminished prefrontal brain function in adults with psychopathology in childhood related to attention deficit hyperactivity disorder. *Psychiatry Research-Neuroimaging* **138**: 157–69.

Faraone SV, Perlis RH, Doyle AE, Smoller JW, Goralnick JJ, Holmgren MA, *et al.* (2005). Molecular genetics of attention-deficit/hyperactivity disorder. *Biol Psychiatry* **57**: 1313–23.

Hebebrand J, Dempfle A, Saar K, Thiele H, Herpertz-Dahlmann B, Linder M, *et al.* (2006). A genome-wide scan for attention-deficit/hyperactivity disorder in 155 German sib-pairs. *Mol Psychiatry* **11**: 196–205.

Klingberg T, Fernell E, Olesen PJ, Johnson M, Gustafsson P, Dahlstrom K, *et al.* (2005). Computerized training of working memory in children with ADHDA randomized, controlled trial. *J Am Acad Child Adolesc Psychiatry* **44**: 177–86.

Lasky-Su J, Anney R, Neale BM, Franke B, Zhou K, Maller, JB., *et al.* (2008). Genome-wide Association Scan of Attention Deficit Hyperactivity Disorder. *Am J Med Gen B: Neuropsychiatric Gen* **147B**: 1337–44.

Linnet KM, Dalsgaard S, Obel C, Wisborg K, Henriksen TB, Rodriguez A, Kotimaa A, *et al.* (2003). Maternal lifestyle factors in pregnancy risk of attention deficit hyperactivity disorder and associated behaviors: Review of the current evidence. *Am J Psychiatry* **160**: 1028–40.

Luman M, Oosterlaan J, Sergeant JA (2005). The impact of reinforcement contingencies on AD/HD: A review and theoretical appraisal. *Clin Psychol Rev* **25**: 183–213.

Madras BK, Miller GM, Fischman AI (2005). The dopamine transporter and attention-deficit/hyperactivity disorder. *Biol Psychiatry* **57**: 1397–1409.

Makris N, Biederman J, Valera, EM, Bush G, Kaiser J, Kennedy DN, *et al.* (2007). Cortical thinning of the attention and executive function networks in adults with Attention-Deficit/Hyperactivity disorder. *Cerebral Cortex* **17**: 1364–75.

McCann D, Barrett A, Cooper A, Crumpler D, Dalen L, Grimshaw K, *et al.* (2007). Food additives and hyperactive behaviour in 3 and 8/9 year old children in the community. *Lancet* **370**: 1560–7.

O'Connor TG, Heron J, Golding J, Glover V (2003). Maternal antenatal anxiety and behavioural/emotional problems in children: a test of a programming hypothesis. *J Child Psychol Psychiatry* **44**: 1025–36.

Oades RD, Sadile AG, Sagvolden T, Viggiano D, Zuddas A, Devoto P, *et al.* (2005). The control of responsiveness in ADHD by catecholamines: evidence for dopaminergic, noradrenergic and interactive roles. *Dev Sci* **8**: 122–31.

Ostrander R, Herman KC (2006). Potential cognitive, parenting, and developmental mediators of the relationship between ADHD and depression. *J Cons Clin Psychol* **74**: 89–98.

Plichta MM, Vasic N, Wolf C, Lesch KP, Brummer D, Jacob C, et al. (2009). Neural hyporesponsiveness and hyperresponsiveness during immediate and delayed reward processing in adult attention-deficit/hyperactivity disorder. *Biol Psychiatry* **65**: 7–14.

Retz WG, Freitag CM, Retz-Junginger P, Wenzler D, Schneider M, Kissling C, *et al.* (2008). A functional serotonin transporter promoter gene polymorphism increases ADHD symptoms in delinquents: Interaction with adverse childhood environment. *Psychiatry Res* **158**: 123–31.

Rubia K, Overmeyer S, Taylor E, Brammer M, Williams SCR, Simmons A, *et al.* (1999). Hypofrontality in attention deficit hyperactivity disorder during higher-order motor control: A study with functional MRI. *Am J Psychiatry* **156**: 891–6.

Rutter M, Beckett C, Castle J, Colvert E, Kreppner J, Mehta M, *et al.* (2007). Effects of profound early institutional deprivation: An overview of findings from a UK longitudinal study of Romanian adoptees. *Eur J Dev Psychol* **4**: 332–50.

Seipp CM, Johnston C (2005). Mother-son interactions in families of boys with attention-deficit/hyperactivity disorder with and without oppositional behavior. *J Abnorm Child Psychol* **33**: 87–98.

Solanto MV, Abikoff H, Sonuga-Barke E, Schachar R, Logan GD, Wigal T, *et al.* (2001). The ecological validity of delay aversion and response inhibition as measures of impulsivity in AD/HD: a supplement to the NIMH multimodal treatment study of AD/HD. *J Abnorm Child Psychol* **29**: 215–28.

Sonuga-Barke EJ, Sergeant J, Nigg J, Willcutt E (2008). Executive dysfunction and delay aversion in ADHD: Nosological and diagnostic implications. *Child Adoles Psychiatric Clin North Am* **17**: 367–84.

Sonuga-Barke EJS, Daley D, Thompson M, Laver-Bradbury C, Weeks A (2001). Parent-based therapies for preschool attention-deficit/hyperactivity disorder: A randomized, controlled trial with a community sample. *J Am Acad Child Adolesc Psychiatry* **40**: 402–8.

Spencer TJ, Biederman J, Madras BK, Faraone SV, Dougherty DD, Bonab AA, *et al.* (2005). In vivo neuroreceptor imaging in attention-deficit/hyperactivity disorder: a focus on the dopamine transporter. *Biol Psychiatry* **57**: 1293–1300.

Taylor E, Rogers JW (2005). Practitioner review: Early adversity and developmental disorders. *J Child Psychol Psychiatry*, **46**: 451–67.

Thapar A, Harrington R, Ross K, McGuffin P (2000). Does the definition of ADHD affect heritability? *J Am Acad Child Adolesc Psychiatry* **39**: 1528–36.

Thapar A, Langley K, Asherson P, Gill M (2007). Gene-environment interplay in attention-deficit/hyperactivity disorder and the importance of a developmental perspective. *Br J Psychiatry* **190**: 1–3.

Valera EM, Faraone SV, Murray KE, Seidman LJ (2007). Meta-analysis of structural imaging findings in attention-deficit/hyperactivity disorder. *Biol Psychiatry* **61**: 1361–9.

Van der Meere J, Marzocchi GM, De Meo T (2005). Response inhibition and attention deficit hyperactivity disorder with and without oppositional defiant disorder screened from a community sample. *Dev Neuropsychol* **28**: 459–72.

Willcutt, EG, Sonuga-Barke, Nigg, JT, & Sergeant, JA (2008). Recent developments in neuropsychological models of childhood psychiatric disorders. In Banaschewski, T & Rohde, LA.(eds) Biological Child Psychiatry: Recent Trends and Developments. *Advances in Biological Psychiatry* **24**: 195–226.

Chapter 4

Assessment

David Coghill and Joseph A. Sergeant

Key points

- ADHD can be assessed with
  - Clinical Interviews
  - Questionnaires and
  - Neuropsychological Measures
- The diagnosis of ADHD is based on clinical judgment of integrated data gathered from multiple sources
- Education of staff at a primary care level, and from education about ADHD is essential to ensure that children with ADHD are promptly identified and referred
- A comprehensive assessment for ADHD is complex and often time consuming. Those conducting these assessments need to be well trained
- The purpose of an "ADHD" assessment is not only to confirm or exclude the presence of ADHD but also to identify whether there are any other problems or disorders that are causing impairment
- At the end of the assessment process the clinician should have developed a comprehensive formulation.

4.1 Introduction

As indicated in Chapter 2, ADHD is a complex disorder wherein the core problems with impairing inattention, hyperactivity, and impulsivity frequently occur alongside other disorders and difficulties (see Box 2.2, Chapter 2). As a consequence the assessment of ADHD symptoms cannot occur in a vacuum and must be considered as part of a comprehensive assessment process. A further complication to the assessment process arises due to the fact that, although there are various tools that can aid assessment, ADHD cannot be diagnosed by using a simple biological test. Rather it involves the integration of information from different sources and a clinical decision making process to resolve conflicting observations and opinions. The diagnosis is however supported by a strong evidence base and there are a range of validated questionnaires and interview schedules to support the assessment process. It is often, but not always, helpful to supplement the information gathered from the child/young person, parents, carers and other family members and teachers with a (neuro)psychological assessment. At the end of the process the clinician will need to determine both a principal and differential diagnosis and make a judgement about the presence of any comorbid disorders.

First we present a brief overview of a series of clinical and neuro-psychological tools that can assist in the evidence based approach to the assessment of ADHD. Following this we present schematically an approach to the assessment process designed to assist the clinician organize their assessments in a structured manner that facilitates good clinical practice and the ongoing evaluation and audit of clinical pathways and processes.

4.2 **Clinical assessment toolkit**

Since ADHD manifests itself behaviourally, three general (complementary) clinical procedures are used to empirically assess the child: interviews, questionnaires, and observations. In this text we present primarily instruments currently used in English speaking countries. Fortunately many of the instruments discussed have been translated into various European and Asian languages. We do however recommend that clinicians wishing to use these international versions first check the data concerning validity and reliability of local versions before use.

4.2.1 **Interview schedules**

Although many clinical assessments will be conducted via a standard clinical history and examination there are occasions where a more structured assessment is useful. In particular clinicians who have not had a full psychiatric or clinical psychology training may find it useful to use a formal interview schedule to guide this part of the assessment process. Two types of interview schedule are available: Structured interview where the questions are fixed and there is an algorithm converting answers into a diagnosis, and the semi-structured clinical interview where the clinician is given a degree of flexibility with respect to the questions asked and then evaluates the respondents answers and reaches a decision as to whether the symptom is present or not. Examples of these two types of interviews are the structured Diagnostic Interview Schedule for Children (DISC-IV; Shaffer, Fisher, Lucas, Dulcan, & Schwab-Stone, 2000), which is based on the Diagnostic and Statistical Manual of Mental disorders, fourth edition (DSM-IV; APA, 1994) and the semi-structured PACS (Taylor et al., 1986). The Development and Well-being Assessment (DAWBA; Goodman 2000) may be of particular interest in some settings as it is possible for parents to complete the interview online and for it to be scored prior to attendance at the clinic for a face to face assessment. A list of commonly used interviews is given in Table 4.1. A need to be able

Table 4.1 Clinical Interviews used in the assessment of ADHD		
Interview	**Full title**	**Reference**
CAPA	Child and Adolescent Psychiatric Assessment	Angold & Costello, 2000
DAWBA	Development and Well-being Assessment	Goodman, 2000
DICA	Diagnostic Interview for Children and Adolescents	Reich, 2000
DISC	Diagnostic Interview Schedule for Children	Schaffer et al., 2000
K-SADS-PL	Schedule for Affective Disorders and Schizophrenia for School-age Children	Kaufman et al., 1997
PACS	Parental Account of Children's Symptoms	Taylor et al., 1986

to account for the differences between the DSM-IV and ICD-10 diagnostic criteria, to be able to extrapolate diagnoses under both sets of rules has led to the development of computer algorithms for easy comparison. The Hypescheme is a good example.

4.2.2 Questionnaires

Questionnaires also fall into two classes: Broadband, that assess for a wide range of psychopathology and allow the clinician to screen for several disorders and; narrow band, which are specific instruments designed to screen for a particular condition. An example of the former is the Child Behaviour Checklist (CBCL, Achenbach, 1991) and of the latter is the Conners Rating Scales (Conners, 1978). Some instruments are multisource (teacher and parent and self respondent) and multidimensional (various types of psychopathology measured) such as the BASC. Questionnaires vary in length, test retest reliability, and the age range originally used to norm to instrument. Careful evaluation of the psychometric properties should be undertaken prior to their use. An overview of several common instruments is presented in Table 4.2.

In clinical practice, it is useful to have a standardized teacher telephone interview to ensure standardized practice. Several tools specifically designed for this purpose are available; (Holmes et al., 2004, Mota & Schachar, 2000). Alternatively, it is possible to use the ADHD-RS as a semi-structured interview (as is frequently done when measuring outcome in clinical trials).

Since children referred for ADHD often present with a considerable variety of associated disorders and deficits, Table 4.3 provides a set of instruments for screening and initial evaluation in these areas. Not all these need to be included as routine but should be used if the information gathered as a part of clinical observation, history taking

Table 4.2 Questionnaires used in the assessment of ADHD		
Abbreviated Title	**Full Title**	**Reference**
Broadband Questionnaires (General Psychopathology)		
CBCL	Child Behaviour Checklist	Achenbach, 1991a
TRF	Teacher Rating Form	Achenbach, 1991b
BASC	Behavioural Assessment System for Children	Reynolds & Kamphaus, 1992
SDQ	Strengths and Difficulties Questionnaire	Goodman, 1997
Narrowband Questionnaires (ADHD)		
CPRS-R CTRS-R	Conners Parent and Teacher Rating Scales - Revised	Conners 1998 a & b; Goyette et al. 1978
ADHD-RS	ADHD Rating Scale - IV	DuPaul et al., 1998
SNAP and SNAP-IV	Swanson, Nolan and Pelham (DSM IV version)	Swanson et al., 1998
SWAN	Strengths and Weaknesses of ADHD—Symptoms and Normal Behavior	Swanson et al., 2005, Hay et al., 2007
SKAMP	Swanson, Kotkin, Atkins, McFlynn & Pelham Scale	Wigal et al., 1998

and evaluation of input from parents, teachers and the child is suggestive of other difficulties. It is however our clinical experience that certain disorders including the pervasive developmental disorders, developmental coordination disorders and dyslexia, whilst common are often missed by the busy clinician and therefore should be considered to be a part of routine assessment process. Further as children with ADHD are assessed both by paediatricians who have not received training in general child psychiatry and mental health practitioners who have not been trained in general developmental assessments each clinician should think about their own strengths and weaknesses and include the appropriate tools in their routine assessment package.

4.2.3 **Observation**

Whilst there are few validated observational measures for ADHD it is our clinical experience that a structured approach to recording observations is often very helpful. In fact although not explicitly an observational measure the SKAMP, that was designed to specifically measure the classroom manifestations of ADHD, has been used

Table 4.3 Questionnaires used to assess for disorders commonly associated with ADHD

Purpose	Title	Reference
Pervasive developmental disorder (PDD)	Children's Social Behaviour Questionnaire (CSBQ)	Hartman et al., 2006
Pervasive developmental disorder (PDD)	Social Communication Questionnaire (SCQ)	Rutter, Bailey and Lord, 2003
Anxiety	Revised Children's Manifest Anxiety Scale (R-CMAS)	Reynolds and Richmond, 1979
Depression	Child Depression Inventory (CDI)	Kovacks, 1985
Mania	Parent version of the Young Mania Rating Scale (P-YMRS)	Gracious et al., 2002
Sleep	Children's Sleep Habits Questionnaire (CSHQ)	Owens et al., 2000
Tics/Tourette's	Tourette's Disorder Scales—Clinician Rated	Storch et al., 2007
Tics/Tourette's	Yale Global Tic Severity Scale	Leckman et al., 1989
Obsessive Compulsive Disorder	Yale-Brown Obsessive Compulsive Scale (Y-BOCS)	Goodman et al., 1989
Coordination disorders/Dyspraxia	Developmental Coordination Disorder Questionnaire (DCD-Q)	Wilson et al., 2000
Language, pragmatics	Children's Communication Checklist	Bishop, 1998
Learning Difficulties Dyslexia Dyscalculia	Woodcock-Johnson III	Woodcock-Johnson, 1989
Dyslexia	Test of Word Reading Efficiency (TOWRE)	Torgesen, Wagner and Rashotte, 1999

to rate observed behaviour in the laboratory school study setting (Wigal, 1998). Within our own clinical teams we have developed a tool to help structure and record their school observations. As this same tool is also used for making observations of children being assessed for pervasive developmental disorders it contains extra information than would not necessarily be required for an ADHD assessment. However we find it helpful to consider both sets of observations for each child even if only to exclude the diagnosis of one or other disorder. Table 4.4 lists the potential domains of interest in a school observation.

Table 4.4 Potential domains of interest in a school observation

General information
- Time of day
- Age of child
- Setting
- Number of children
- Number of adults
- Activity (e.g. math's class, quiet time, group or individual working, etc.)
- Room type and set up (e.g. traditional class room, open plan, individual or group desks, etc.)

Observed behaviours
- Overactivity (e.g. out of seat, climbing, fidgeting, etc.)
- Impulsivity (e.g. answering questions directed at others, butting in, shouting out, unable to wait, etc.)
- Inattention (e.g. needs reminding to stay on task, difficulty getting started, poor task completing, etc.)
- Oppositional behaviours (argues with teacher or peers, aggressive to others, etc.)
- Evidence of mood lability
- Level of communication and interaction with others
- Ability to use comprehend and use language
- Ability to socially interact with others
- Reciprocal social interactions
- Repetitive behaviours
- Ability to imitate others
- Ability to play appropriately
- Evidence of anxiety

Figure 4.1 Summary of current meta-analytic evaluations of commonly employed neuropsychological tests and tasks for ADHD—Typically Developing children comparison

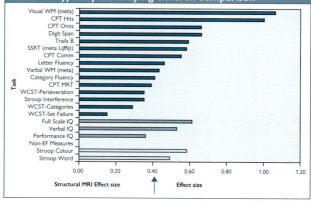

4.2.4 **Neuropsychological assessment**

Neuropsychological assessments cannot prove or disprove the presence of ADHD they can however support the clinical assessment and add valuable information about an individual's cognitive specific strengths and weaknesses which can help shape management plans and strategies.

4.2.5 **Neuropsychological discrimination between ADHD and typically developing children**

At a time where the providers of health services have to justify any additional examinations that are used, it is helpful to consider the extent to which the main dimensions of neuropsychological functioning are able to discriminate between ADHD and typically developing children. For this purpose, Figure 4.1 details the effect sizes associated with several of the executive function (EF) measures and compare these with non-EF measures and findings derived from standardized IQ assessment as in the WISC III or WAIS. An arrow indicates the comparative strength of structural magnetic resonance imaging to perform the same discrimination (Valera et al., 2007). This suggests that both working memory and vigilance give the strongest discrimination. This Figure also indicates that a non-Executive Function, colour naming in the Stroop, is more power than some EF measures (e.g. WCST set failure) suggesting that for assessment purposes, both executive and non-executive functions need to be considered. Several important measures are not included in this Figure; measures of Delay aversion, have an effect size of 0.66 (Willcutt et al., 2008) and of non-executive visuospatial memory effect size 0.89–0.92 (Rhodes et al., 2005). It is however important to point out that due to the heterogeneity inherent to ADHD many children with ADHD will still perform well on these tasks and not everybody with poor performance will have ADHD.

4.2.6 **Neuropsychological assessment as an adjunct to clinical assessment**

When it is considered appropriate to conduct more extensive neuropsychological examination a wide range of potential tasks can be considered. Table 4.5 provides an overview of cognitive domains that the clinician and neuropsychologist are most likely to wish to evaluate. The Table also includes examples of some (but not all) of the readily available tests/tasks that have been found to be helpful assessing these domains in clinical practice. Performance on these tasks can help inform clinicians and teachers about potential obstacles to learning and suggest strategies for managing them. In particular the identification of short term memory problems and slow processing speed can be of particular help to both parents and teachers. For example a child with memory problems will do better with written rather than verbal instructions and when instructions are given in small chunks rather than all together.

Table 4.5 Neuropsychological Domains and Tests/Tasks

Domain	Neuropsychological Test/Task
Attention	Stroop Task
	Freedom from Distractibility (WAIS-R)
	Letter Cancellation Task
Vigilance/Sustained Attention	Continuous Performance Task (time on task)
Inhibition	Stop Signal Reaction Time Task
	Opposite Worlds (TEACH)
Planning	Tower of London / Hanoi, Stockings of Cambridge
Fluency	F-A-S Fluency test
Flexibility	Trails B
	Wisconsin Card Sorting Test
Working Memory	Self Ordered Pointing Task, CANTAB Spatial Working Memory
	Digit Span Forwards and Backwards
	Corsi Block Pointing, CANTAB Spatial Span
	CANTAB Delayed Matching to Sample

4.3 The assessment process

Having a clearly thought through and comprehensive assessment protocol that covers all the right territory is as, if not more, important as having the appropriate tools (see Box 4.1).

Box 4.1 Process Diagrams

We have designed a series of process diagrams, based on the recommendations made in the European Guidelines for the Assessment and Treatment of ADHD (Taylor et al., 2004). These will be used here to illustrate an approach to developing a comprehensive care pathway for the recognition and assessment of ADHD. Each diagram describes; a trigger, the clinicians involved, the aims, European Guidelines recommendations and the expected outcomes. This approach will be continued in Chapter 7 "Organizing and Delivering Treatment".

These process diagrams should not be seen as prescriptive and we suggest that they are used to stimulate discussion within teams and services and to help problem solve any barriers to practice and to develop an evidence based care pathway that works for their particular circumstances.

4.3.1 **Recognition**

The assessment process actually starts before a referral to specialist services is made with the identification in the family, school and/or community that a child is having difficulties and that these difficulties may be due to ADHD. Whilst this may sound simple, it is the case that across much of the world, with the possible exception of the USA and certain European countries such as the Netherlands and Germany, only a very small minority of those children with ADHD are currently receiving a diagnosis. For example a recent audit of ADHD care in Scotland identified that only 0.6% of children are currently diagnosed as suffering from ADHD compared to epidemiological projections of between 3 and 5% (i.e. between 80 and 90% of children are currently not diagnosed). Further research from the UK suggests that the major stumbling block to recognition is a failure by primary care doctors to recognize that the problems presented to them by parents are an indication of possible ADHD.

At this stage in the process it is essential that the primary care physician listens to and believes the parents descriptions of behavioural difficulties and recognizes the importance of the core ADHD symptoms of inattention, hyperactivity and impulsivity (see Box 4.2). It is also important for them to be able to distinguish these symptoms from those other disorders such as oppositional defiant disorder, pervasive developmental disorder, mental retardation, hearing impairment, or restless leg syndrome. Whilst screening for ADHD in the general community is not recommended it is appropriate for the primary

Box 4.2 Recognition of ADHD	
Trigger	• Parent or Teacher expresses ADHD related concern
Clinicians involved	• Primary care
Aims	• Detect symptoms • Distinguish from other disorders
European guidelines recommentdations	• Parent questionnaires (e.g. SDQ, Connors) • Teacher information • Physical examination • Check Hearing
Outcomes	• If ADHD symptoms are present and resulting in social impairment refer to a Child and Adolescent Mental Health Service (CAMHS) or if not available to developmental or behavioural paediatrics

care and education staff to be trained in the use and interpretation of common questionnaires such as the broadband SDQ and narrow-band Conners' questionnaires. Good communication between health and education staff is very helpful but often difficult at the primary care level, however school reports are a valuable source of collateral information about a child's difficulties and their use should be encouraged. A physical examination is also essential to exclude physical causes for the child's difficulties.

Primary care staff will generally have had very little education about ADHD and it is therefore important that specialist services consider how they can facilitate learning both here and in educational settings to ensure increased recognition of ADHD and appropriate referral to specialist services for a fuller assessment.

4.3.2 **Assessment**

As with any other mental health assessment the primary aim of the "ADHD" assessment is to develop a formulation that fully explains the child/young person's difficulties (Box 4.3). If the assessment is to successfully meet this aim several key points need to be borne in mind. In order to meet criteria for ADHD it is not enough that the patient is assessed as having the requisite number of symptoms. It is also necessary that these symptoms are developmentally inappropriate, pervasive across more than one setting, that they are associated with a significant degree of impairment, and that they cannot be accounted for by an alternative explanation. It is also necessary to consider, and assess for a wide range of possible comorbid or coexisting disorders including both psychiatric and non-psychiatric disorders (e.g. dyslexia, developmental coordination disorder and hearing problems).

As a consequence a full assessment for ADHD is never a simple task and requires skill, specialist training and experience with a broad range of mental health and developmental disorders and is often best conducted by members of a multidisciplinary team. Ideally such a team will include (or at least have good access to) mental health, paediatric, clinical/neuro-psychological, and occupational therapy skills, and have access to speech and language therapy, family/systemic therapy, physiotherapy and educational skills. It is also the case that a full assessment takes time and it is not usually possible to complete a full assessment in a single meeting. *Whilst the full assessment must be seen as a whole most of these recommendations can be broken down into several key "tasks".*

The basis for assessment consists of patient's history, observation of the patient's current behaviour and the account of parents and teachers about the child's functioning in his/her places. There is often poor agreement between informants (children, parents, and teachers) about the child's mental health. Children often do not reliably inform about their own behavioural symptoms and have low test-retest agreement for ADHD symptoms. They can however make invaluable comments about other aspects of their life and their inner worlds. Parents seem to be good informants with respect to ADHD symptoms but often are less accurate at describing emotional difficulties.

Teachers have a tendency to overestimate the presence of ADHD symptoms, especially when another disruptive behavioural disorder is also present. With adolescents, the value of the information given by teachers is often much less, as they have several teachers each of

Box 4.3 **Assessment of ADHD**	
Trigger	• Child/young person is referred with possible ADHD
Clinicians involved	• Child and Adolescent Mental Health Services (CAMHS) • Developmental/behavioural paediatrics
Aims	• To assess whether or not patient meets diagnostic criteria for ADHD • To distinguish ADHD from other disorders and exclude other explanations for behaviours • To assess whether patient is suffering from any comorbid disorders
European guidelines recomendations	• A full assessment should be conducted. This will require more than one meeting and should include: • Clinical interview with the parents • A separate interview with the child • Preshool, Kindergarten and school information • School observation and investigations • Intelligence/cognitive tests if there is a specific indication
Outcomes	• Confirmation or exclusion of an ADHD diagnosis • In cases where ADHD is confirmed there should also be confirmation or exclusion of any comorbid disorders • In cases where a diagnosis of ADHD is excluded there should be a formulation of an alternative explanation for the presentation.

whom spends little time with each class, which prevents them from knowing each student well enough to comment accurately. However the process of diagnostic evaluation necessarily involves collection of data from each of these sources as each can provide complementary information.

4.3.2.1 *Clinical interview with the parents*

This forms the core of the clinical assessment (Table 4.6). Tasks can be divided into a general evaluation of the child, their problems and the context within which they are occuring and specific questioning about ADHD and its common comorbidities.

Whilst these lists make the distinction between the two tasks seem very clear and orderly it is important to remember that parents will often have waited a long time to tell their story "to someone who understands" and at the same time may be quite anxious about the assessment process. It is therefore very important that they are allowed space and time to describe the difficulties from their perspective and to vent their frustrations. The assessment can be seen as the start of a relationship between the clinical services and the family and as those with a diagnosis of ADHD will often require a prolonged period of treatment it is important to get off on the right foot and start to cultivate a strong therapeutic alliance from the beginning. This will pay dividends down the line where continued concordance and compliance with treatment is likely to be central to success.

An assessment of possible parental ADHD is also an important facet of the assessment process. Parents with unrecognized and untreated ADHD can find it much more difficult to parent their children and have been demonstrated to make less use of parent training packages.

Past clinical history of behaviour is essential for diagnostic definition, since only a small number of patients present the characteristic signs and symptoms of ADHD at the assessment appointments. The absence of symptoms at the office does not rule out the diagnosis. These children often have some ability to control the symptoms voluntarily, or during activities in which they are greatly interested. Therefore, many times, they can spend hours in front of the computer or videogame, but cannot spend a few minutes in front of a book in the classroom or at home.

A detailed social and family history is of paramount importance. Clinicians should pay attention to family history of ADHD, perinatal history, since various studies have found a higher prevalence of ADHD in preterm babies and low birth weight infants. Careful follow-up of this risk group is important for the early identification of signs and symptoms that may indicate a possible diagnosis of ADHD.

Table 4.6 Clinical interview with the parents

General Evaluation

- Clarify presenting complaints
- Make systematic evaluation of symptoms
- Describe how problems developed
- Developmental history including previous professional reports
- Family history of ADHD
- Pregnancy and birth history (foetal growth, toxaemia, bleeding or severe infections during pregnancy, maternal diabetes or epilepsy, other maternal illness or traumas, poor maternal nutrition, maternal medication, nicotine, alcohol and drug use, gestational age, birth complications, birth weight, neonatal complications)
- Early developmental history (milestones for psychomotor development, language, attachment, sleep and feeding problems, growth and early temperament)
- Medical history (especially tics and epilepsy, psychosis—if adolescent)
- Medication (especially anticonvulsants, antihistamines, sympathomimetics, steroids)
- Family functioning and family problems
- Social networks and other resources

Specific Questioning

- The behaviours that comprise ICD-10 HKD and DSM-IV ADHD diagnoses, including:
  - Their relationship to current level of development
  - Any situational variation
  - Ages of onset
  - Development over time
  - Their presence in other family members
- A rating of impairment
- Related problems (e.g. behavioural and learning problems, emotional problems, tics, conduct disorder, alcohol problems)
- Parent completed rating scales

45

As described in section 4.2 the use of standardized interview schedules and scales like the SNAP-IV and ADHD-RS to identify the signs and symptoms of ADHD is widely accepted, although many clinicians do not yet employ them on a routine basis.

4.3.2.2 *Separate interview with the child*

This is usually more helpful in addressing general adjustment and comorbidity than for assessing the presence or absence of diagnostic criteria which are usually more accurately described by parents, family members, teachers and other observers (Table 4.7).

With respect to the observation of ADHD behaviours within the clinic setting it is important to remember that children with ADHD, just like their healthy counterparts, will often moderate their behaviours in novel settings. It is therefore not uncommon for these children, who are described as perpetually "on the go" by their parents, to appear well controlled for the first few clinic appointments. This should not usually be used as evidence against the presence of ADHD. It is however often very useful to make an assessment of the child's language skills, social relatedness and ability to use imagination as this may provide pointers towards (or away from) a pervasive developmental disorder.

Table 4.7 Separate interview with the child

Should focus on:
- Functioning in the family, the school and the peer group
- A general evaluation of psychopathology (especially emotional problems and self esteem)
- The child's attitude to, and coping with, their disorder.

Self report rating scales may be helpful as an adjunct to an interview (especially for detecting emotional problems)

Observation of behaviour during the interview can be useful especially if ADHD or other behavioural problems are observed. However a negative observation does not mean problems are not present and repeated observation is often required. An observer should focus on assessing:
- The presence of social disinhibition
- Ability to concentrate and persist
- Any evidence of language disorder.

4.3.2.3 *Preschool, kindergarten and school information and school observations*

Information from school is essential for the diagnosis of ADHD. This can be gathered in various ways (Table 4.8). In our clinical practice we always ask for copies of all previous school reports and of any specific assessments that have been conducted within the school setting as well as a contemporaneous structured written report addressing current academic attainments, behavioural difficulties and interpersonal relationships.

Table 4.8 Preschool, kindergarten and school information

Obtain information from teacher about:
- Behaviour and behaviour problems
- Development
- Social functioning
- Situational variation in behaviour and symptoms that may indicate comorbid or differential diagnoses.

Standardized questionnaires can help to obtain a broad coverage of information (e.g. SDQ , CBCL and Conners')

Further written or telephoned reports may also be needed:
- For a full view of the child at school
- To assess the coping style of the teacher
- The teacher child relationship.

Where necessary a structured telephone interview to clarify the presence/absence of ADHD symptoms and impairments is conducted with the class teacher using one of the instruments described above. If there is still doubt about the diagnosis or other aspects of functioning a school observation is conducted focusing on the behaviours described previously in section 4.2.3 and Table 4.4, the interactional and coping style of the teacher and the teacher child relationship.

4.3.2.4 *Physical evaluation and investigations*

The physical evaluation is an important part of the assessment process and can also provide essential baseline measurements for the treatment phase. Clinical audit suggests that this is the part of the assessment most frequently missed out (especially in mental health settings) and therefore particular attention should be paid to the recommendations described in table 4.9 when developing or reviewing care pathways. On the other hand physical investigations (other than height, weight, head circumference, pulse and blood pressure) are not routinely required and their use should be guided by the history and physical examination (see Table 4.9).

4.3.2.4 *Intelligence and cognitive testing*

The routine assessment of intelligence is not required for all cases. It can however be very helpful, for example where there is a suspicion of a mild to moderate cognitive impairment or learning disorder (mental retardation). In such cases it is important to distinguish behaviours indicative of ADHD from those that are associated with delayed development. We are aware that lack of time and resources often restrict a clinician's ability to ask for intelligence testing but testing should always be considered when there is any problem related to classroom adjustment or progress. When time is scarce, a brief assessment of verbal performance (e.g. in the UK the British Picture Vocabulary Scale, BPVS) or the short Wechsler Abbreviated Scale of Intelligence (WASI) or equivalent is better than no assessment.

The neuropsychological heterogeneity inherent to ADHD (not all children with ADHD will necessarily have any one particular neuropsychological deficit) and the lack of specificity between particular tasks and particular psychiatric disorders (for example ADHD, pervasive developmental disorders and schizophrenia are all associated with deficits in a range of executive functions) result in problems of sensitivity and specificity for neuropsychological tasks in the diagnostic assessment of ADHD. However the identification of a neuropsychological deficit known to be associated with ADHD can be helpful in supporting a clinical diagnosis. Cognitive testing can also be of great assistance in helping to characterize strengths and weaknesses

Table 4.9 Physical evaluation and investigations

Physical evaluation

Height, weight and head circumference should always be recorded.

Pulse and blood pressure (especially if considering medication).

General examination is always needed and should include:

- An assessment of general physical health,
- Any evidence of poor standards of care/abuse,
- Stigmata of congenital disorders (e.g. Foetal alcohol syndrome, Williams syndrome, neurofibromatosis),
- Vision check (Snellen chart),
- Hearing check; in the UK and many European countries all children should already have had proper audiology testing. The assessing clinician should check whether this has happened and refer for audiometry if it has not.
- Evidence of neurodevelopmental immaturity in gross and fine motor functions,
- Screen for motor and vocal tics.

Investigations

These should not be routine but guided by history and physical examination:

- Where there is any evidence for compromised cardiac function an ECG should be carried out,
- Where there is a history suggestive of seizures an EEG should be carried out,
- If there is a developmental delay, chromosome estimation and a DNA assessment for Fragile X should be conducted,
- Audiograms are required if clinical evaluation has not ruled out significant hearing loss.

Brain scanning is not required unless there is a particular reason to suspect a brain lesion.

of patients and/or the presence of comorbid disorders like dyslexia and mental retardation. In particular the identification of short term memory problems and slow processing speed are of practical help to teachers.

4.3.3 Diagnosis and formulation

Following the collection of information from the various sources this needs to be integrated and a judgment made regarding diagnosis. Clinical training, skill and experience are often required to reconcile conflicting information. The aim is to make a full formulation with diagnosis, differential diagnosis, a description of any predisposing, precipitating and perpetuating factors, acknowledgement of any comorbid or coexisting disorders and a description of any complicating factors (e.g. peer relationship problems, bullying, high expressed emotion at home, poverty etc.). In cases where further treatment will be offered it is also helpful to integrate a formulation of the symptoms and problems that will be the focus of treatment (see Table 4.10 and Chapter 7).

Table 4.10 Potential target symptoms and problems

- Core ADHD symptoms
- Oppositional and disruptive behaviour in the home
- Oppositional and disruptive behaviour in the classroom
- Academic problems
- Peer group relationships
- Other associated symptoms (e.g. anxiety, mood instability, depression, dyspraxia, speech and language problems etc.).

References

Achenbach TM. (1991a). *Manual for the child behaviour checklist.* Burlington, VT: Department of Psychiatry, University of Vermont.

Achenbach TM. (1991b). *Integration guide for the 1991 CBCL-4-18, YSR, and TRF profiles.* Burlington, VT: Department of Psychiatry, University of Vermont.

American Psychiatric Association. (1994). *Diagnostic and statistical manual of mental disorders* (4th ed.). Washington, DC: Author.

Angold A, & Costello EJ. (2000).The Child and Adolescent Psychiatric Assessment (CAPA). *Journal American Academy Child Adolescent Psychiatry* **39**: 39–48.

Bishop DV. (1998). Development of the Children's Communication Checklist (CCC): a method for assessing qualitative aspects of communicative impairment in children. *Journal Child Psychology & Psychiatry*, **39**: 879–91.

Conners CK, Sitarenios G, Parker JD, Epstein JN. (1998a). Revision and restandardization of the Conners Teacher Rating Scale (CTRS-R): factor structure, reliability, and criterion validity. *Journal Abnormal Child Psychology* **6**: 279–91.

Conners CK, Sitarenios G, Parker JD, Epstein JN. (1998b). The revised Conners' Parent Rating Scale (CPRS-R): factor structure, reliability, and criterion validity. *Journal Abnormal Child Psychology* **26**: 257–68.

Curran, S., Newman, S., Taylor, E., & Asherson, P. (2000). Hypescheme: An operational criteria checklist and minimum data set for molecular genetic studies of attention deficit and hyperactivity disorders. *American Journal of Medical Genetics* **96**: 244–50.

DuPaul, G.J., Power, T.J., Anastopolous, A.D., & Reid, R. (1998). *ADHD Rating Scale–IV: Checklists, norms, and clinical interpretation.* New York: Guilford Press.

Fristad MA, Weller RA, Weller EB. (1995). The Mania Rating Scale (MRS): further reliability and validity studies with children. *Annals Clinical Psychiatry* **3**: 127–1232.

Goodman, R. (1997). The strengths and difficulties questionnaire. *Journal Child Psychology & Psychiatry* **38**: 581–6.

Goodman WK, Price LH, Rasmussen SA *et al.* (1989). The Yale-Brown Obsessive Compulsive Scale. I. Development, use, and reliability. *Archives General Psychiatry* **46**: 1006–11.

Goyette CH, Conners CK, Ulrich RF. (1978). Normative data on revised Conners Parent and Teacher Rating Scales. *Journal Abnormal Child Psychology* **6**: 221–36.

Gracious BL, Youngstrom EA, Findling RL, Calabrese JR. (2002) Discriminative validity of a parent version of the Young Mania Rating Scale. *J.Am.Acad.Child Adolesc.Psychiatry* **41**(11): 1350–1359.

Hartman, C. A., Luteijn, E., Serra, M., & Minderaa, R. (2006). Refinement of the children's social behaviour questionnaire (CSBQ): an instrument that describes the diverse problems seen in milder forms of PDD. *Journal of Autism and Developmental Disorders* **36**: 325–42. doi:10.1007/s10803-005-0072-z.

Hay DA, Bennett KS, Levy F, Sergeant J, Swanson J. (2007). A twin study of attention-deficit/hyperactivity disorder dimensions rated by the strengths and weaknesses of ADHD-symptoms and normal-behavior (SWAN) scale. *Biological Psychiatry* **61**: 700–5.

Holmes J, Lawson D, Langley K *et al.* (2004).The Child Attention-Deficit Hyperactivity Disorder Teacher Telephone Interview (CHATTI): reliability and validity. *Br. J. Psychiatry* **184**: 74–8.

Kaufman J, Birmaher B, Brent D, Rao U, Flynn C, Moreci P, Williamson D, Ryan N. (1997). Schedule for Affective Disorders and Schizophrenia for School-Age Children-Present and Lifetime Version (K-SADS-PL): initial reliability and validity data. *Journal American Academy Child Adolescent Psychiatry* **36**: 980–8.

Kovacs M. (1985). The Children's Depression, Inventory (CDI). *Psychopharmacological Bulletin* **21**: 995–8.

Leckman JF, Riddle MA, Hardin MT, Ort SI, Swartz KL, Stevenson J, Cohen DJ. (1989). The Yale Global Tic Severity Scale: initial testing of a clinician-rated scale of tic severity. *Journal American Academy Child Adolescent Psychiatry* **28**: 566–73.

Mota, V.L., & Schachar, R.J. (2000). Reformulating attention-deficit/hyperactivity according to signal detection theory. *Journal American Academy Child & Adolescent Psychiatry* **39**: 144–1151.

Owens JA, Spirito A, McGuinn M. (2000). The Children's Sleep Habits Questionnaire (CSHQ): psychometric properties of a survey instrument for school-aged children., **23**(8): 1043–51.

Reich W. (2000).Diagnostic interview for children and adolescents (DICA). *Journal American Academy Child Adolescent Psychiatry* **39**: 59–66.

Reynolds, C.R., & Kamphaus, R.W. (1992). *Behavioral assessment system for children (BASC)*. Circles Press, MN: AGS.

Reynolds CR, & Richmond BO. (1979). Factor structure and construct validity of "what I think and feel": The Revised Children's Manifest Anxiety Scale. *Journal Personality Assessment* **43**: 281–3.

Rhodes SM, Coghill DR, Matthews K. (2005) Neuropsychological functioning in stimulant-naive boys with hyperkinetic disorder. *Psychol. Med.* **35**(8): 1109–20.

Rutter, M., Bailey, A., & Lord, C. (2003). The social communication questionnaire manual. Los Angeles: Western Psychological Services. Social Communication Questionnaire (SCQ).

Shaffer D, Fisher P, Lucas CP, Dulcan MK, Schwab-Stone ME. (2000). NIMH Diagnostic Interview Schedule for Children Version IV (NIMH DISC-IV): description, differences from previous versions, and reliability of some common diagnoses. *Journal American Academy Child Adolescent Psychiatry* **39**: 28–38.

Storch EA, Murphy TK, Geffken GR, Sajid M, Allen P, Roberti JW, Goodman WK. (2005). Reliability and validity of the Yale Global Tic Severity Scale. *Psychological Assessment* **17**: 486–91.

Storch EA, Merlo LJ, Lehmkuhl H, Grabill KM, Geffken GR, Goodman WK, Murphy TK. (2007). Further psychometric examination of the Tourette's Disorder Scales. *Child Psychiatry Human Development* **38**: 89–98.

Swanson J, Schuck S, Mann M, Carlson C, Hartman K, Sergeant J, *et al* (2005). Categorical and dimensional definitions and evaluations of symptoms of ADHD: The SNAP and the SWAN Ratings Scales [Draft]. Available at: http://www.adhd.net/SNAP_SWAN.pdf. Accessed May 25, 2005.

Taylor, E., Schachar, R., Thyorley, G., & Wieselberg, M. (1986). Conduct disorder and hyperactivity: I. Separation of hyperactivity and antisocial conduct in British child psychiatric patients. *British Journal of Psychiatry* **149**: 760–7.

Torgesen, J.K., Wagner, R.K., & Rashotte, CA. (1999). *Test of Word Reading Efficiency*, Austin, TX: Pro-Ed, Inc.

Valera EM, Faraone SV, Murray KE, Seidman LJ. (2007). Meta-analysis of structural imaging findings in attention-deficit/hyperactivity disorder, **61**, 1361–9.

Willcutt, E.G., Sonuga-Barke, Nigg, J.T., & Sergeant, J.A. (2008). Recent developments in neuropsychological models of childhood psychiatric disorders. In Banaschewski, T. & Rohde, L.A. (eds) *Biological Child Psychiatry: Recent Trends and Developments. Advances in Biological Psychiatry* **24**: 195–226.

Wigal SB, Gupta S, Guinta D, Swanson JM. (1998).Reliability and validity of the SKAMP rating scale in a laboratory school setting. *Psychopharmacological Bulletin* **34**: 47–53.

Wilson,B.N., Kaplan,B.J., Crawford,S.G., Campbell,A., and Dewey,D. (2000). Reliability and validity of a parent questionnaire on childhood motor skills. *American Journal Occupational Therapy* **54**: 484–93.

Woodcock, R.W., & Johnson, M.B. (1989). *Woodcock-Johnson Psycho-Edcuational Battery-Revised*. Allen. Tx: DLM Teaching resources.

Chapter 5

Pharmacological treatments

Alessandro Zuddas

Key points

- Drug treatment should be based on a comprehensive assessment and diagnosis including full medical history and physical examination
- It should always be part of a comprehensive treatment plan that includes psychological, behavioural, and educational advice and interventions.
- Methylphenidate, amfetamines, and atomoxetine, are effective treatments via distinct neurochemical mechanisms. They should be used as main options for the management of ADHD in children and adolescents
- Drug treatment should be closely monitored for both common and unusual (but potentially severe) side effects.

5.1 **Approach to treatment**

Any treatment plan for ADHD must be based on a comprehensive diagnostic evaluation: the clinician should document that the child meets the criteria for a diagnosis of an ADHD subtype, being aware of possible concomitant medical or psychiatric conditions or learning disabilities (see Chapter 4 "Assessment"). Rather than focusing just on the disorder, the child should be treated as an individual in her/his particular social context. Before starting treatment, it is important to identify (and quantify) the target outcomes for guiding therapy decisions during treatment. Depending on individual circumstances, both psychosocial intervention ("behaviour modification") and pharmacotherapy can be considered, (see chapters 6 "Psychosocial and other non-pharmacological treatments" and 7 "Organizing and delivering treatment"), as potential first treatments for children and adolescents with ADHD (Taylor et al., 2004; NICE, 2008).

Stimulant medications—dexamfetamine or methylphenidate (MPH)—and atomoxetine (ATX) are the most effective psychopharmacological treatments for ADHD. Racemic amfetamine is the oldest stimulant preparation used to treat ADHD since the seminal observations of Bradley in 1937; although more potent than MPH, amfetamine is less used in Europe and is not commercially available in many countries. However, recently an amfetamine pro-drug (lisdexamfetamine) has been licensed in the US and is under consideration for approval in Europe and in other parts of the world. The use of MPH for the treatment of ADHD is well established and has been reviewed by EUNETHYDIS for European Child and Adolescent Psychiatry (Taylor et al., 2004, Banaschewski et al., 2006). MPH is licensed in the US and in most European countries as part of comprehensive treatment programmes in children (over 6) and adolescents. Different extended release formulations have been developed. More recently, a patch formulation (transdermal) has been approved in the US. ATX is the only non-stimulant medication officially approved for the treatment of ADHD. It has a license for children and adults in the USA, for children and for adults if their treatment has started in childhood in Europe.

5.2 **Molecular mechanism of action of ADHD medications**

After synaptic release, monoamines (norepinephrine, dopamine and serotonin) are taken up by specific active membrane transport proteins (Norepinephrine transporter–NET, Dopamine transporter- DAT, serotonin transporter–SERT, respectively) and, when in the cytoplasma, by specific vesicular transporter proteins (Vesicular Monoamine Transporter 2; VMAT-2) into the synaptic vesicle. MPH, amfetamines, and ATX are effective via distinct neurochemical mechanisms.

5.2.1 **Amfetamines**

Racemic amfetamine contains equal amounts of d- and l-amfetamine isomer. The amfetamine d-isomer (dextroamfetamine) inhibits reuptake via both membrane transporters and, at higher concentration, vesicular transporters. D-amfetamine also increases basal DA and NE release by binding to the vesicular monoamine uptake 2-transporter (VMAT2) and inducing reverse transport through the plasma membrane into the cytoplasma. In vitro, affinity of d-amfetamine is higher for NET (in prefrontal cortex) than for DA (in the striatum), and much lower for serotonin. The amfetamine l-isomer is less potent (13-fold) than the d-isomer in inhibiting the accumulation of DA or NA into vesicles, and 5–7 times less potent in inhibiting the synaptic membrane transport (Easton et al., 2006).

Box 5.1 From molecular mechanism to clinical effects

Stimulants increase extracellular levels of dopamine (DA) and norepinephrine (NE) by blocking the respective monamine transporters (amfetamines also increase catecholamine release from synaptic vesicles). Exactly how these actions relate to the stimulant effects on attention and performance is, however, still unclear. DA and NE decrease background firing rate of neurons, thus increasing noise-to signal ratio. During cognitive tasks methylphenidate (MPH) has been shown to increase cerebral blood flow (CBF) in dorso-lateral prefrontal and posterior parietal cortices in healthy controls (Metha *et al.*, 2000) and in the prefrontal cortex in adults with ADHD (Schweitzer *et al.*, 2004); it appears to decrease metabolic activation of task-irrelevant brain regions, thus focusing activation and improving performance (Volkow *et al.*, 2008).

5.2.2 **Methylphenidate**

MPH is 40- and 70-fold less potent than *d*-amfetamine at inhibiting vesicular accumulation of DA or NA, but a similarly potent inhibitor of synaptic re-uptake of DA, and a slightly less potent inhibitor of NE re-uptake. Racemic MPH consists of both *d*- and *l*-threo-enantiomers in a 50/50 ratio. The *d*-threo-enantiomer is pharmacologically more active than the l-threo-enantiomer (10-fold for norepinephrine reuptake; 10- to 40-fold for dopamine reuptake (Heal & Pierce, 2006).

5.2.3 **Atomoxetine**

ATX is a selective inhibitor of the synaptic reuptake of NE. *In vitro*, ATX does not directly modulate DA transporter synaptic uptake or DA or NE vesicular transport. However, *in vivo* ATX specifically increases extracellular levels of DA in the prefrontal cortex but not the striatum probably by modulating the cortical synaptic DA uptake via the NE transporter (Swanson *et al.*, 2006).

A summary of the molecular mechanisms of atomoxetine and other medications for the treatment of ADHD is shown in Figure 5.1.

5.3 **Pharmacokinetics and interaction with other drugs**

5.3.1 **Amfetamines**

Absorption of amfetamine is fast, with peak plasma levels occurring about 3 hours after oral administration. Food does not affect total absorption, but does delay it. Metabolism is through the liver. Children eliminate amfetamine faster than adults, the elimination life of d-amfetamine being about 1 hour shorter in 6–12 year old children

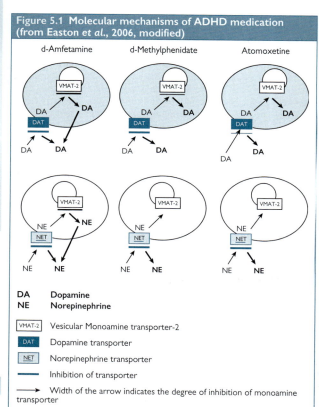

Figure 5.1 Molecular mechanisms of ADHD medication (from Easton *et al.*, 2006, modified)

d-Amfetamine	d-Methylphenidate	Atomoxetine

DA	Dopamine
NE	Norepinephrine

VMAT-2	Vesicular Monoamine transporter-2
DAT	Dopamine transporter
NET	Norepinephrine transporter
—	Inhibition of transporter
⟶	Width of the arrow indicates the degree of inhibition of monoamine transporter

(average 9 hours) than in adults (average about 10 hours). Acidification of urines increases urinary excretion of amfetamines. Ingestions of acidic substances such as ascorbic acid, or fruit juices, may lower absorption, whereas gastrointestinal alkalinizing agents, such as sodium bicarbonate, seem to increase absorption.

5.3.1.1 *Onset and duration of action*

Consistent with the pharmacokinetics profile, the onset of action of amfetamines is rapid, within 1 hour after administration. For immediate release preparations, the duration of action is around 4–5 hours, which is longer than for MPH, but still requires at least b.i.d. administration to ensure adequate coverage.

Mixtures of different d-dexamfetamine and l-dexamfetamine salts formulated for immediate or modified release are available in the United States but not in Europe (Adderall). Adderall XR$^{®}$ (Shire) 20 mg provides comparable plasma concentrations to Adderall immediate release 10 mg bid administered 4 hours apart. Its administration results in ascending plasma levels of amfetamine up to a peak at about 7 hours after dosing. This is followed by a gradual decline that results in low but detectable plasma levels 24 hours after dosing.

5.3.1.2 *Lisdexamfetamine*

Lisdexamfetamine is dextroamfetamine that has been covalently attached to the essential amino acid, L-lysine. Following oral administration, the amide linkage between the two molecules is enzymatically hydrolyzed in the gastrointestinal tract, thus releasing active dextroamfetamine. Lisdexamfetamine itself is not pharmacodynamically active and neither does it result in high dextroamfetamine levels when injected or snorted, and thus it is likely to have a lower abuse potential compared to conventional stimulants. Lisdexamfetamine appears to have efficacy and tolerability comparable to other extended-release stimulant formulations used to treat ADHD, but reduced potential for abuse-related liking effects (Faraone, 2008).

5.3.1.3 *Interaction with other drugs*

Amfetamine may potentiate stimulating effects of other drugs on the cardiovascular or central nervous system.

5.3.2 Methylphenidate

Oral MPH is rapidly absorbed from the gastrointestinal tract, with peak plasma concentrations occurring about 1.5–3 hours after administration. Food delays the time to maximum plasma concentration from 1.5 hours when fasting to 2.5 hours after heavy breakfast: it is usually recommended to give the medication just before breakfast. MPH is primarily metabolized through de-esterification to ritalinic acid, which has no clinically significant pharmacological activity and is excreted in the urine. Dl-*threo*-methylphenidate undergoes enantioselective metabolism in the liver, which results in marked differences in the plasma concentrations of its isomers. The elimination plasma steady half-life of *d-threo*-methylphenidate is about 3–3.5 hours. Because of this short-half life, steady state is never achieved during treatment and there is no carry over from one day into the next. Metabolism and pharmacokinetics are similar in school-age children and adults.

5.3.2.1 *Extended release preparations*

Laboratory school studies suggest a close relationship between pharmacokinetics (PK) and pharmacodynamic (PD) properties. Optimal clinical effect appears associated with increasing plasma levels across the day: preparations with bimodal release systems ensure an initial sharp plasma peak occurring about 1.5 hours after dosing, followed by a second peak several hours later followed by a gradual decline. Ritalin LA® (Novartis), Concerta® XL (Janssen-Cilag) Equasym XL® (UCB/Shire), and Medikinet Retard® (Medice) all provide a mixture of immediate and extended-release MPH; they differ in the mechanics of the delayed-release system and in the proportion of immediate release to delayed release methylphenidate. Figure 5.2 shows the PK profile over time of these different formulations; the actions on behaviour parallel the concentrations in the blood. Concerta® XL action lasts about 12 hours, Equasym XL®, Ritalin LA® and Medikinet Retard® lasts between 6 and 8 hours.

Different delivery profiles provide the clinician with increased options when choosing which preparation to use for a particular patient, as well as a more flexible and sensitive individualized adjustment whilst retaining the benefits of an ER preparation. It should be noted however, that PK profiles may show considerable inter-individual variation. Caution should be observed when generalizing from aggregated profiles to individual patient cases. The onset of action, in particular, can be delayed or may be attenuated in the afternoon, requiring the concomitant administration with a low dose of immediate release preparation.

Figure 5.2 MPH and amfetamine plasma levels over time with different preparations and their IR/ER proportions

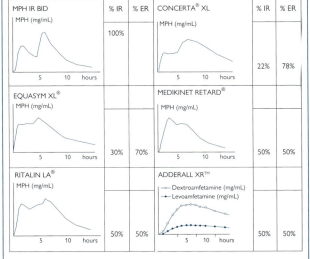

Figure 5.2 is reproduced from Banaschewski *et al.* (2006) with kind permission from Steinkopff, Heidelberg.

Recently a transdermal system that delivers racemic MPH through the skin directly into the bloodstream has been developed and is available in the US. Racemic MPH is solubilized in acrylic in very high concentrations and mixed with adhesive to form concentrated pockets of drug. The concentration gradient results in an efficient diffusion of the drug out of the adhesive layer. Reproducible plasma concentrations within the same patient have been demonstrated, with intra-subject coefficients of variation of approximately 20%. With a 9-hours wearing time of the system the time-course of clinical effectiveness was from 2 to 12 hours after skin application. Plasma concentrations, and probably efficacy, decline rapidly after patch removal. Since first-pass liver metabolism is avoided, the ratio of *l-* versus *d-threo*-methylphenidate concentration is significantly higher than after oral administration.

5.3.2.2 *Interaction with other drugs*

MPH has little interference with the metabolism and pharmacokinetics of other drugs. It can inhibit the metabolism of anticonvulsants such as phenobarbital, phenytoin and primidone, and of some antidepressants (tricyclics, SSRIs). MPH can also interact with other drugs that also have a sympathomimetic effect, causing tachycardia, tremor, and nervousness more likely than either drug given in isolation.

Four cases of sudden death were reported in children with ADHD taking concurrent administration of MPH and clonidine, but no causal links between MPH treatment and cardiovascular adverse events or the occurrence of ECG abnormalities have been established (Tourette's Syndrome Study Group, 2002).

5.3.3 **Atomoxetine**

ATX is metabolized mainly through the hepatic cytochrome P450 2D6 enzymatic system (CYP2D6) resulting in metabolites with clinically significant activity. About 5–10% of Caucasians and 2% of African Americans have genetically determined low CYP2D6 activity ("poor metabolizers"). In poor metabolizers, plasma levels of ATX can be 10-fold higher compared to subjects with normal CYP2D6 activity ('extensive metabolizers'). Mean elimination half-life is about 22 hours in poor metabolizers compared to 5 hours in extensive metabolizers. At steady state the duration of brain NET inhibition appears to be longer than ATX plasma levels are detectable; once daily ATX is associated with a decrease of 3,4-dihydroxyphenylethylene glycol (DHPG), which is the main brain metabolite of norepinephrine and a biomarker of central NET inhibition, persisting for at least 24 h. Interestingly, there also appears to be a dissociation between the pharmacokinetic and pharmacodynamic profiles for ATX with evidence that even after once-daily dosage the clinical effects of ATX can last throughout the day.

The onset of clinical effectiveness of ATX is slower than that of stimulants: as for tricyclic antidepressants (see section 5.6.4), it may vary between 2 and 4 weeks (and possibly longer in some individuals).

5.3.3.1 *Interaction with other drugs*

Concomitant administration of fluoxetine or paroxetine, drugs that inhibit the CYP2D6 activity, results in higher plasma levels of ATX. Likewise, slower metabolism of ATX and higher plasma levels should be expected during concomitant use of other drugs that inhibit the CYP2D6 system Although there are case reports in the literature and despite it having become common practice in some countries to combine ATX with stimulants where there appears to be a lack of treatment response with mono-therapy, it must be noted that there has been no systematic investigation of concomitant use for this combination or for ATX with any other drug for the treatment of ADHD. In particular safety data is lacking for this combination. Possible interactions between ATX and other drugs for ADHD treatment have not been systematically studied.

5.4 **Clinical efficacy**

5.4.1 **Short term efficacy**

5.4.1.1 *Stimulants*

There is substantial evidence supporting the efficacy and effectiveness of stimulants (MPH in particular) in reducing ADHD symptoms over treatment periods up to a year and in doses up to 60 mg daily. Numerous placebo-controlled randomized control trials confirm the substantial short-term benefit (SIGN 2001, Banaschewski *et al.*, 2006, NICE 2008). Stimulants reduce restlessness, inattentiveness and impulsiveness markedly and rapidly. Effect sizes on hyperactivity symptoms are typically between 0.8 and 1.1. The response rate to stimulants is at least 70% and, if non-responders are treated with the second stimulant, the cumulative response rate is at least 95% (Efron *et al.* 1997). The corresponding numbers needed to treat (NNT; a measure of outcome, see Box 5.2) are between 3 and 5. Stimulants have also been documented to improve the quality of social interactions, decrease aggression and increase compliance. Patients with ADHD and comorbid anxiety or disruptive disorders have as robust a response of their ADHD symptoms to stimulants as do patients who do not have these comorbid conditions: MPH effects on anxiety or oppositional defiant behaviour *per se* are, however, controversial. Nevertheless, taking stimulants, the hyperactive child is rated by peers as more co-operative, greater fun to be with, and is more likely to be considered to be a best friend. Medication may not enhance the hyperactive child's social judgement or eliminate their negative perceptions of their peers; a longer period of treatment may be required to counteract the negative reputation of a hyperactive child and to eliminate social deficits.

Medication usually starts with immediate release MPH, beginning at a low level e.g., 5–10 mg (depending on age and weight of the child) in a single daily dose or bd or tds, and should be monitored collecting information from parent and teachers using simple rating scales (see Section 7.3.3 "Initiating a new medication"). The dose should be titrated until either a good clinical response; or the maximum dose is reached (0.7 mg/kg/dose up to three times a day, i.e. a total daily dose of 2.1 mg/kg/day [or in rare cases: 1.0 mg/kg/dose, if dose is given twice daily, i.e. a total daily dose of 2.0 mg/kg/day]—subject to a ceiling of 100 mg/day for immediate release, or the equivalent modified-release dose); or adverse effects appear—whichever comes first. The total daily dose should be administered in divided doses. Three daily doses are recommended, but practical considerations may dictate a twice daily regime (e.g. at breakfast and lunch). Adult patients are variable in their dosage requirement, and up to 1.0 mg/kg/dose, or even 2 mg/kg daily has been used. The most common dose range used in European adult ADHD clinics for IR methylphenidate is 10–20 mg taken 3–5 times daily, with both higher and lower dosing required in individual cases. Our suggested maximum is 30 mg for each dose (Taylor *et al.*, 2004). The dosages given are different to British National Formulary (BNF) and children's BNF and Summary of Product Characteristics. Monitor closely for side effects. Long acting preparations may be considered to start treatment (see Chapter 7 for a fuller account of titration protocols).

5.4.1.2 **Atomoxetine**

ATX has been shown to be effective in decreasing hyperactivity, impulsivity and inattention in school-age children with ADHD as compared with placebo with an effect size on hyperactivity symptoms of around 0.7 and NNT (see Box 5.2) of around 4 (Banaschewski *et al.*, 2006). The treatment effect can be clinically evident at the end of the first week of treatment, but full therapeutic activity may not emerge until after 2–6 weeks of treatment and in some cases may require even longer. The therapeutic benefit persists in time and is not subject to attenuation or tolerance.

ATX has been shown effective in reducing symptoms of both ADHD and comorbid anxiety, with a moderate effect size (0.5) for anxiety, relative to placebo. ATX has been shown a useful alternative in treatment-emergent or comorbid tics since it does not worsen tics and may even improve them (see also Box 5.3). Because of his lack of abuse potential, ATX has also been suggested as primary drug of choice in adolescents with ADHD and comorbid Substance Use Disorder. ATX use as first choice medication in specific patient populations is discussed in Chapter 7.

Box 5.2 Improvement and Normalization: Effect size & NNT

The calculation of effect sizes standardizes the magnitude of the difference in improvement (change) in drug and placebo groups so that a 1-point difference indicates that the active treatment and placebo groups differ by 1 standard deviation on a particular outcome measure. This allows a direct comparison of treatment effectiveness across studies, including those that have used different outcome measures. A commonly used effect size index is the standardized mean difference [SMD: the difference in outcome scores between drug and placebo groups divided by the pooled standard deviation (of the placebo and medication group at end of treatment)].

The actual outcome may be better characterized by the concept of normalization and measured by the Numbers Needed to Treat (NNT). Normalization rates are defined as the proportion of patients normalized, e.g., having no problems more than "mild" (i.e. Conners scale T-score < 63 or SNAP < 1/item). The NNT corresponds to the expected number of patients needed to be treated to see one patient normalize in terms of symptoms with medication and would not have normalized on placebo therapy.

Effect sizes and NNTs for medications to treat ADHD are better than those reported for most other psychiatric drugs. For example, the effect sizes and NNT for antidepressants to treat adult depression or obsessive-compulsive disorder are about 0.5 and 9, respectively, and for atypical antipsychotics to treat schizophrenia around 0.25 and 20 (Banaschewski *et al.*, 2006).

5.4.2 **Long-term efficacy of stimulants and efficacy of combination with psychosocial intervention**

The long-term and distal effects of stimulants have been less well investigated, primarily because it is extremely difficult to run controlled studies for years. Thus, it remains unclear if successful control of ADHD symptoms during childhood results in better prognosis in adult years. One large-scale, random allocation, non-blind trial in the USA focused on the comparison between careful medication management, intensive behaviourally oriented psychosocial therapy, a combination of the two, or a simple referral back to community agencies (which usually resulted in medication) (MTA Cooperative Group, 1999). The main conclusions after 14 months' treatment were that careful medication was more powerful than behaviour treatment, and considerably more effective than routine medication in the community. The superiority of careful medication to behaviour therapy was particularly striking because behaviour therapy provision was much more intensive and prolonged than could be achieved by a community service.

Box 5.3 Approach to common adverse events during stimulant treatment	
Adverse event	**Possible approach**
Loss of Appetite (es. No food intake at lunch)	1. If early in treatment, look for possible tolerance over time to this side effect 2. Decrease dose, if clinically possible 3. Increase caloric intake at breakfast and dinner. 4. Monitor weight
Loss of weight	1. Decrease dose (unless child is overweight). 2. Increase caloric intake at breakfast and dinner; add caloric snacks in between; allow late evening meal 3. Consider lower dose or no medication during weekend 4. Monitor weight: tolerance to this effect often develops.

Early insomnia (difficulty falling asleep)	1. If immediate release prep.: allow no dosing after 3 pm.
	2. If extended release prep.:
	  a. reduce dosing,
	  b. change formulation or
	  c. start treatment early in the morning and give medication before breakfast (more rapid absorption).
	3. Be sure that there is an appropriate bedtime routine (e.g., reading).
	4. Consider atomoxetine.
	5. Add evening dose covering bedtime

Blunted affect ("zombie"-like appearance)	1. Decrease dose, if possible. 2. Try different preparation 3. Consider atomoxetine
Tics (new onset)	1. Discontinue treatment and see if tics go away. 2. Restart treatment and see if tics come back. 3. Consider atomoxetine

There were many advantages in adding medication to behaviour therapy, but relatively few to adding behaviour therapy to medication. The combination of behaviour therapy and medication did have some benefits: better control of aggressive behaviour at home; improving the overall sense of satisfaction of parents; possibly reducing the medication dosage; increasing the "normalization" rate (reduction of problems to an average level of minor and below).

The follow-up at 36 months, 22 months after ending the active treatment phase of the study, at which point parents and children were free to choose the actual treatment, showed that all four original groups had a similar outcome, respectively improvement by comparison with pre-treatment baseline scores. Various explanations are possible: the effects of more intensive therapy disappear when the intensive treatment is stopped; self-selection of patients to treatments at the end of the randomization phase may lead to similar outcome (many children assigned to behavioural intervention started medication, but a significant percent of those on intensive drug management during the first 14 months of the study, actually withdrew medication during the follow-up). The most favourable overall development was found in children who had been initially randomized to the MTA medication regime, whether or not they were taking medication at 36 months suggesting some lasting benefit for some children with ADHD. (The reader is referred to Section 7.4 for treatment monitoring issue).

5.4.3 **Relapse prevention by atomoxetine**

In children and adolescents who had responded favourably to an initial 12-week, open-label period of treatment with ATX, ATX was superior to placebo in maintaining response for a subsequent 9 months period which was conducted under double-blind conditions. Interestingly, only 50% of the subjects randomized to placebo relapsed to baseline severity (Michelson, 2004). Following 1 year of treatment with ATX, continued treatment over the following 6 months was associated with superior outcomes compared with blinded discontinuation with placebo substitution, but the magnitude of symptom relapse after drug discontinuation was often relatively modest, suggesting that subjects treated for a year with good results should be reassessed for their need for ongoing drug treatment (Buitelaar *et al.* 2006).

5.5 **Safety**

5.5.1 **Stimulants and substance abuse**

Stimulants are drugs of potential abuse. In animal models, both MPH and amfetamine display features typical of substances of abuse, such as compulsive self-administration, with neglect of other activities, including food intake. There are, however, important differences between therapeutic use and non-therapeutic abuse of stimulants that involve doses, route of administration and social context. When abused, stimulants are typically injected or snorted with rituals of self-administration, powerful conditioning and at doses that are much higher than therapeutic doses in search of euphoria. For MPH, the reinforcing effects and "high" are associated with the rapid changes in serum concentrations, and presumably rapid dopamine increases, associated with intravenous injection or insufflation, whereas the therapeutic effects are associated with slowly ascending serum concentrations and presumably smoothly rising dopamine levels found after oral administration. Euphoria is practically unknown among medicated children.

Concern has been raised that therapeutic use of stimulants may result in "sensitization" and possibly increase the risk for substance abuse later in life. However, ADHD itself, associated with impulsivity, often impaired social judgment, and conduct disturbances, is a risk factor for substance abuse. Disentangling whether treatment of ADHD with stimulants results in a decrease (or an increase) in substance abuse in early adulthood in randomized clinical trials is practically impossible. Naturalistic follow-up studies do not support the contention that stimulant treatment increases risk for substance abuse (e.g., Mannuzza et al., 2008).

Stimulant medication prescribed for the treatment of ADHD can however be diverted by patients or families toward abuse (Wilens et al., 2008). Thus, history of substance abuse or the presence of current substance abuse in the family can, depending on the precise situation be seen as either a relative contraindication for stimulant prescription, especially in the immediate release preparation, or as a reason for extremely close monitoring of a patient's stimulant use. The extended release formulations of stimulants are less prone to diversion because these preparations cannot be easily crushed into powder for injection or snorting, and also because the once-a-day administration makes parental supervision easier to enforce. Non stimulant medications (i.e. atomoxetine) are another option for these patients.

5.5.2 Adverse events of stimulant medication

The common adverse effects of MPH include decreased appetite, sleep disturbance, headaches, stomach aches, drowsiness, irritability, tearfulness, mildly increased blood pressure and pulse. Rare but more severe adverse events can include psychotic symptoms and sensitivity reactions requiring discontinuation of the medication.

Thus, stimulants are contraindicated in several circumstances, most of them uncommon in childhood: schizophrenia, severe depression, hyperthyroidism, cardiac arrhythmias, moderate to severe hypertension, angina pectoris, glaucoma, hypersensitivity, and concomitant use—or use within the last 2 weeks—of monoamine oxidase (MAO) inhibitors. Caution is advised in: patients with motor tics, patients with known drug dependence or history of drug dependence, anorexia nervosa, or a history of suicidal tendency and during pregnancy or breast-feeding.

Strategies for dealing with side effects include monitoring, dose adjustment of the stimulant, adjustment in the timing of doses, switching medication, and, less commonly, adjunctive pharmacotherapy to treat the side effects (Taylor et al., 2004, Banaschewski et al., 2006).

5.5.2.1 *Weight and growth*

Treatment with stimulants causes dose-related reductions in expected height and weight (Swanson *et al.*, 2007, Faraone *et al.*, 2008). Beside decreased food intake, weight gain can also be suppressed by increased activity and metabolic shifts (e.g., increased fat mobilization). These mechanisms can be related to direct medication effects or secondary to changes in neuroendocrine hormone secretion: stimulants increase dopaminergic activity which in turn may inhibit GH secretion. Some studies also suggest that growth dysregulation may be an epiphenomenon of ADHD rather than a cause of its treatment, but more work is needed to confirm that hypothesis and to draw conclusions about the impact of long-term stimulant treatment on final adult height. A recent systematic review indicated that reductions in expected height and weight are, on average, small and appear to attenuate with time: nevertheless it is essential that physicians monitor for growth deficits to identify those children who will require a change in their medication regimen (Faraone *et al.*, 2008).

5.5.2.2 *Tics and Tourette's syndrome*

While Tourette's syndrome was once considered an absolute contra-indication to stimulants more recently several studies have shown that stimulants are quite effective in controlling ADHD in the context of Tourette's disorder and they do not inevitably worsen motor or vocal tics (Tourette's Syndrome Study Group, 2002). Stimulants may be considered as an appropriate treatment option for children with ADHD and tic disorders, but careful monitoring during treatment is required: if the tics worsen, the stimulant should be suspended. It is critical to document the type and severity of tics before starting treatment in order to establish a baseline against which to assess treatment-associated changes.

5.5.2.3 *Pulse and blood pressure*

MPH may have a small but clinically non-significant effect (average increase <5mmHg) on blood pressure and lead to a slight increase in pulse rate (average <5bpm).

5.5.2.4 *Seizures and epilepsy*

Although longer-term effects of MPH and its effects in children with frequent seizures need to be studied, current evidence supports the use of MPH for the treatment of ADHD in those patients whose seizures are under control (Torres *et al.*, 2008). When epilepsy is poorly controlled, frequency of seizures should be carefully monitored: if their frequency increases, or seizures develop de novo, then MPH should be stopped. Dexamfetamine may be an alternative.

5.5.2.5 *Sleeplessness*

It is clinically important to distinguish children whose insomnia is an adverse drug effect from those children whose insomnia may be due to the recurrence—or worsening—of behavioural difficulties as the medication effect subsides. For the first group of children, reducing the last dose of the day may be sufficient. For the latter group, an evening dose may be helpful.

5.5.2.6 *Other Contraindications for stimulants*

Presence of florid psychosis or mania is a contraindication to the use of stimulants, which can worsen these symptoms by stimulating the dopaminergic transmission. In well-controlled bipolar disorder, use of stimulants for comorbid ADHD can be considered on an individual basis in combination with appropriate antimanic treatment.

5.5.3 **Adverse events of atomoxetine**

Common adverse effects associated with ATX include abdominal pain, nausea and vomiting, decreased appetite with associated weight loss, dizziness, and slight increases in heart rate and blood pressure. These effects are normally transient and may not require discontinuation of treatment. ATX can increase blood pressure and heart rate. At a group level, these changes appear of little clinical significance, but there is individual variability and the clinicians should measure vital signs before starting treatment and then periodically (at least monthly first, then at least quarterly) afterwards.

Very rarely, liver toxicity, manifested by elevated hepatic enzymes and bilirubin with jaundice, has been reported. Out of 351 spontaneous reports, three cases of reversible drug-induced liver injury were deemed probably related to the drug (Bangs *et al.*, 2008). Six more cases have been more recently reported by FDA (FDA, 2009). Patients and caregivers should be alert to signs and symptoms of liver failure throughout ATX treatment: ATX should be discontinued and not resumed if a patient presents with jaundice or laboratory evidence of hepatotoxicity. Seizures are a potential risk for ATX. Suicide-related behaviour (suicide attempts and suicidal ideation) has been reported. In double-blind clinical trials, suicide-related behaviours occurred at a frequency of 0.44% in ATX-treated patients (one case of attempted suicide and five of suicidal ideation). As for stimulants, treatment with ATX can be associated with decreased appetite and weight loss.

5.5.4 **Severe cardiovascular effects of ADHD medication**

In 2006 the US FDA conducted a review on reports of sudden death in patients treated with ADHD medications using data from their Adverse Event Reporting System (AERS).

The review identified 14 paediatric and 4 adult sudden death cases reported with MPH between January 1992 and February 2005. None of them appears solely or directly related to MPH. Six of the 14 paediatric sudden deaths occurred in children with structural cardiovascular abnormalities that likely preceded the use of MPH.

The safety review found seven cases of sudden death with ATX (three children and four adults) of which one had lymphocytic myocarditis and two had toxic levels of olanzapine or a possible seizure preceding death; none of these patients had prior history of cardiovascular problems or cardiovascular structural abnormalities. The review reported that none of the cases appears solely or directly attributable to ATX at therapeutic doses. The cases were highly confounded. None of the patients had structural cardiovascular abnormalities.

The review concluded that the rate of sudden death with MPH and ATX was below background rates available. No definitive conclusions can be drawn from the analyses of AERS cases due to the inherent limitations of the AERS and uncertainty regarding information on drug utilisation and background incidence of sudden death.

Also the EMEA's Committee for Medicinal Products for Human Use (CHMP) has recently reviewed MPH due to concerns over cardiovascular risks (hypertension, heart rate increases, and arrhythmias) and cerebrovascular risks (migraine, cerebrovascular accident, stroke, cerebral infarction cerebral vasculitis, and cerebral ischaemia). After reviewing all available data, the Committee concluded that there was no need for an urgent restriction to the use of MPH-containing medicines, but that new recommendations on prescribing and on pre-treatment screening and ongoing monitoring of patients are needed to maximize the safe use of these medicines (EMEA, 2009). Specific recommendations are reported in the Boxes 5.4 and 5.5.

For a recent extensive review on adverse events of ADHD medications see also Graham & Coghill, 2008.

5.6 **Other drugs**

5.6.1 **Clonidine**

Clonidine is an alpha 2–receptor agonist that down-regulates adrenergic transmission, thus causing hypotension and other effects of decreased autonomic sympathetic activity. Clonidine acts on the brain with sedative and anti-anxiety effects. It is marketed for the treatment of hypertension, but also used off label for the treatment of ADHD in children and, in adults, for the management of symptoms of withdrawal from drug of abuse.

The evidence for efficacy of clonidine to treat ADHD is weaker than that for stimulants and ATX, and thus far , does not univocally support its efficacy. Evidence for its efficacy to reduce tics in children with ADHD and tic disorder is better. In children comorbid for ADHD and Tourette, a randomized controlled study comparing clonidine, MPH and placebo, clonidine appeared to be most helpful for impulsivity and hyperactivity; MPH for inattention. The proportion

Box 5.4 Precautions before starting medications

Drug treatment for children and young people with ADHD should always form part of a comprehensive treatment plan that includes psychological, behavioural and educational advice and intervention, full mental health and social assessment

Pre-medication screening should include:
- full history and physical examination, including:
  - assessment of history of exercise syncope, undue breathlessness and other cardiovascular symptoms
  - heart rate and blood pressure (plotted on a percentile chart)
  - height and weight (plotted on a growth chart)
  - family history of cardiac disease and examination of the cardiovascular system
- an electrocardiogram (ECG) if there is past medical or family history of serious cardiac disease, a history of sudden death in young family members or abnormal findings on cardiac history or examination (e.g. of syncope or undue breathlessness on exercise)
- risk assessment for substance misuse and drug diversion (where the drug is passed on to others for non-prescription use).

Box 5.5 Precautions during treatment

- Height and weight of treated patients should be monitored and compared to age-matched norms
- Blood pressure and heart rate should be monitored regularly. Any problems that develop should be investigated promptly.
- Medications (ATX in particular) should be discontinued in patients with jaundice or laboratory evidence of liver injury and should not be restarted.
- The use of stimulants or ATX could cause or worsen some psychiatric disorders such as depression, suicidal thoughts, hostility, psychosis, and mania. All patients should be carefully screened for these disorders before treatment and monitored regularly for psychiatric symptoms during treatment
- There is a relative lack of information on the long-term effects of MPH. For patients who take medications for more than a year, doctors should interrupt treatment at least once a year to determine whether continued treatment is necessary.

of individual subjects reporting a worsening of tics as an adverse effect was no higher in those treated with MPH (20%) than those being administered clonidine alone or placebo (22%). Compared with placebo, measured tic severity lessened in all active treatment groups in the following order: clonidine + MPH, clonidine alone, MPH alone. (Tourette's Syndrome Study Group, 2002).

Clonidine has prominent cardiovascular and central nervous system effects that lower blood pressure and can result in symptoms of orthostatic hypotension, such as dizziness, palpitations, and rapid heart beat, upon standing. Bradycardia is a possible side effect. Other common side effects include dry mouth and sedation.

The sedative effect of clonidine has been used to induce sleep in children with early insomnia, either idiopathic or consequent to use of stimulant medication. While this practice is apparently not uncommon in some communities, no adequate testing of its potential benefit and harms has been conducted.

5.6.2 **Guanfacine**

The alpha-2 adrenergic receptor agonist guanfacine, which is pharmacologically similar to clonidine but has a longer duration of action and less sedating activity, has been more recently introduced to treat ADHD. An extended release preparation was found to be effective in ameliorating ADHD symptoms in children and adolescents. The most frequent adverse events include somnolence, headache, fatigue, sedation, dizziness, irritability, upper abdominal pain, and nausea, which usually emerge within the first 2 weeks of treatment and then remit spontaneously during treatment. Considerations about cardiovascular effects are similar as for clonidine (Sallee *et al.*, 2008).

5.6.3 **Bupropion**

Bupropion is an antidepressant, has been shown to be better than placebo in decreasing ADHD symptoms in children. Its efficacy is however smaller than that of stimulants. The mechanism of action of bupropion remains unclear: it is a weak inhibitor of the presynaptic reuptake of norepinephrine, dopamine and serotonin. It is rapidly absorbed with plasma peak at about 2 hours and has a plasma elimination half-life of 8–24 hours (mean 14 hours) in adults. Drug interactions are possible due to its extensive liver metabolism.

Bupropion can cause nausea, insomnia, and palpitations; it can also trigger tics and cause dermatological reactions, such as rash and urticaria, at times severe enough to lead to discontinuing the drug. Bupropion increases the overall risk for seizures, but this effect is very small if the dose is maintained within 300 mg/day. The possible effect of age on the risk for seizures has not been investigated.

5.6.4 **Tricyclics**

Tricyclics constitute the first generation of antidepressants: they were introduced in the 1960s and remained the usual treatment of mood and anxiety disorders in adults until the introduction of the selective serotonin reuptake inhibitors in the late 1980s. Some of them have been tested also in the treatment of ADHD in both children and adults. Imipramine, desipramine, nortriptyline, amitriptyline and clomipramine have been found to be more effective than placebo for the control of ADHD symptoms, but in general less effective than stimulants.

None of them has been approved by the FDA or EMEA for the treatment of ADHD: they were prescribed off-label for children with ADHD, but after the introduction of atomoxetine, they are rarely used for concerns about their potential toxicity, cardiovascular in particular. Sudden and unexplained deaths have been reported in children receiving therapeutic doses of tricyclic, most often desipramine. Some of these cases followed strenuous physical exercise. While a cause-effect relationship between therapeutic doses of tricyclic and sudden unexplained death has not been proven, the use of tricyclics has much declined after these reports. If treatment with a tricyclic is undertaken, careful pretreatment assessment and monitoring during treatment is necessary. In addition, parents should be informed of the potential risks and advised to keep the prescribed medication in a safe place away from child's reach.

Tricyclics inhibit the presynaptic norepinephrine reuptake. They have also antimuscarinic activity, which is responsible for some of their side effects such as dry mouth, constipation, tachycardia, and sedation, and quinidine-like effects, which are responsible for delayed electrical conduction in the heart and related potential cardiotoxicity. Blood pressure is sometime increased due to adrenergic stimulation.

Tricyclics are metabolized by hepatic microsomal enzymes, primarily the CYP2D6. On average, metabolism tends to be faster in children than in adults because of the greater hepatic parenchyma relative to body mass during development. The elimination plasma half-life of imipramine can range from 6 to 24 hours and that of desipramine from 12 to 76 hours in adults. Nortriptyline pharmacokinetics was studied in children and its elimination plasma half-life was found to range from 11 to 42 hours in 5–12 years old and from 14 to 89 in 13–16 years old.

5.6.4.1 *Approach to treatment with tricyclics*

The tricyclic whose efficacy in ADHD has been best documented is desipramine. It is however unfortunate that most of the sudden deaths were associated with therapeutic doses of desipramine (in spite of the wider use of imipramine; for these reasons Desipramine is contra-indicated in the UK). It should be noted that desipramine is an active metabolite of imipramine, and that administration of imipramine results in plasma levels of desipramine. Despite the numerous unknowns about tricyclics and cardiotoxicity, it may be prudent, if a tricyclic is to be used at all, to consider imipramine or nortriptyline ahead of desipramine.

Before starting treatment, the child should receive a complete physical examination with ECG recording. Treatment should be considered only if the following limits are not exceeded on the ECG:

200 msec for the PR, 120 msec for the QRS, and 450 msec for the QTc, and the heart rate should be regular and not higher than 100 bmp. If there is personal history of arrhythmias, dizziness, fainting, palpitation, or heart abnormalities, a more thorough evaluation by a cardiologist is appropriate. Family history of sudden unexpected death or life threatening arrhythmias should be reason for avoiding use of tricyclic medication.

The starting dose for imipramine is usually about 10-25 mg once a day, then gradually raised in a few days to b.i.d. and further adjusted based on clinical effects and side effects. Clinical effects can become evident in a few days, but full response may take weeks and the dose usually needs multiple adjustments. The usual therapeutic dose is between 0.7 and 3.5 mg/kg/day. The ECG, pulse, and blood pressure are to be monitored when a steady state is reached (usually after 4–5 days of treatment) and each time the dose is increased above 3 mg/kg/day. Dosages for other tricyclics are similar. Abrupt discontinuation of tricyclic treatment can trigger withdrawal symptoms, such as nausea, vomiting, headache, lethargy, flu-like symptoms. To prevent withdrawal symptoms, the medication must be tapered off gradually, decreasing the dose by 10–25 mg every 2–3 days until complete discontinuation.

5.6.4 Modafinil

Modafinil is a "wakefulness-promoting agent", it is marketed for the treatment of narcolepsy and has been occasionally used for the management of inattention in adults. Its mechanism is not clear (i.e. non-dopaminergic activating action on frontal cortex) but unrelated to the sympathomimetic stimulants. Cases of Steve-Johnson's syndrome were reported during clinical trials in children, leading the FDA to require new large randomized controlled trials: there is currently not enough data to consider modafinil an effective and safe medication for ADHD.

5.7 Special Populations

5.7.1 Preschoolers

Most treatment research in ADHD has been conducted in children of 6-10 years of age. The official label of MPH warns that this drug is not approved for use under age 6. Since amfetamine is an older drug and the label information reflects the lower regulatory standards 50 years ago, it is approved for use down to age 3 years. A recently completed, publicly funded, multi-site trial (Preschoolers with ADHD Treatment Study PATS, Greenhill et al., 2005) randomizing 160 children younger than 6 years to placebo or IR MPH 1.25, 2.5, 5 mg, or 7.5 mg t.i.d found that the magnitude of the MPH effect (at 2.5–7.5 mg dose range) was somewhat lower than typically observed in school-aged children. MPH presented the typical profile of side effects of stimulant medication in older children, but the frequency and severity of adverse events (i.e., mood lability) were greater and led to treatment discontinuation in about 9% of cases. Continuous treatment for about 9–10 months was associated with a slight but detectable decrease in height and weight growth (Swanson *et al.*, 2007).

5.7.2 Children with Autism or Other Pervasive Developmental Disorders (PDD)

According to the current nosological system, a formal diagnosis of ADHD is not possible in the context of autism or other PDD. However, children with these severe developmental disorders often suffer from hyperactivity, inattention and impulsiveness that cause substantial impairment in their ability to learn and interact with others. A multisite trial of MPH immediate release 7.5–25 mg/day given with t.i.d. dosing in children with autism or other PDD and significant ADHD symptoms indicate that this medication is effective in reducing ADHD symptoms severity but only in about 50% of the cases, a rate that is substantially lower than that observed in non-PDD children with ADHD. The rate of children unable to tolerate the side effects of MPH is correspondingly higher (18%) compared with normal children (less than 5%). MPH can be considered for children with prominent ADHD symptoms in the context of autism or other PDD, but its relatively low efficacy and tolerability must be taken into account. A few open label studies with ATX have begun to show some efficacy, but further studies are required.

5.7.3 Adults

In the US, all classes of medication approved for use in children are also effective and approved for the treatment of adults with ADHD. However, in Europe, none of these medications is licensed for use in adults with ADHD in Europe, except for ATX which is licensed for the continued treatment of adults who have been started on this medication in childhood or adolescence.

While the number of drug trials in adults is far smaller than in children, the results of these trials have consistently demonstrated the effectiveness of stimulants to reduce the level of ADHD symptoms in adults fulfilling diagnostic criteria for ADHD. Treatment regimes in adults are similar to those used in children, although higher doses might be necessary.

A recent meta-analysis including 22 placebo-controlled trials (n = 2,203) suggests a relative benefit in terms of clinical response for shorter-acting stimulants, primarily immediate release MPH, which was 3.26 times greater than for longer-acting stimulants and 2.24 times greater than for longer-acting forms of bupropion. Neither non-stimulants nor longer-acting stimulants reduced adverse effects compared to shorter-acting stimulants. Immediate release MPH was also the only drug shown to reduce ADHD symptoms in adults with substance abuse disorders (Peterson *et al.*, 2008).

In considering these findings, however, it should be taken in account that the studies considered in the meta-analysis had different aims and design, that data on academic, occupational and social functioning, cardiovascular toxicity, and longer-term outcomes, influences of ADHD subtype and/or comorbidities, and misuse/diversion were lacking and that comorbidity with substance use disorder should be considered as an important contraindication for the use of short acting stimulants.

As for adolescents, in adults with ADHD and comorbid with substance use disorder, atomoxetine or stimulant formulations with a reduced potential for abuse (i.e. osmotic micropumps or microbeeds as in Concerta® XL or Ritalin LA®, Equasym XL®, Medikinet Retard®, respectively) should be considered as first choice medications.

References

Banaschewski T, Coghill D, Santosh P, Zuddas A, Asherson P, Buitelaar J, Danckaerts M, Dopfner M, Faraone SV, Rothenberger A, Sergeant J, Steinhausen HC, Sonuga-Barke EJ, Taylor E (2006). Long-acting medications for the hyperkinetic disorders: A systematic review and European treatment guideline. *Eur Child Adolesc Psychiatry* **15**: 476–95.

Bangs ME, Jin L, Zhang S, Desaiah D, Allen AJ, Read HA, Regev A, Wernicke JF (2008). Hepatic events associated with atomoxetine treatment for attention-deficit hyperactivity disorder. *Drug Saf.* **31**(4): 345–54.

Buitelaar JK, Michelson D, Danckaerts M, Gillberg C, Spencer TJ, Zuddas A, Faries DE, Zhang S, Biederman J (2007).A randomized, double-blind study of continuation treatment for attention-deficit/hyperactivity disorder after 1 year. *Biol Psychiatry* **61**(5): 694–9.

Easton N, Steward C, Marshall F, Fone K, Marsden C (2007). Effects of amfetamine isomers, methylphenidate and atomoxetine on synaptosomal and synaptic vesicle accumulation and release of dopamine and noradrenaline in vitro in the rat brain. *Neuropharmacology* **52**(2): 405–14.

Efron D, Jarman F, Barker M (1997) Methylphenidate Versus Dexamfetamine in Children With Attention Deficit Hyperactivity Disorder: A Double-blind, Crossover Trial, *Pediatrics* **100**: e6.

European Medicines Agency (2009). EMEA makes recommendations for safer use of Ritalin and other methylphenidate-containing medicines in the EU. http://www.emea.europa.eu/pdfs/human/referral/methylphenidate/2231509en.pdf

FDA (2009). http://www.fda.gov/CDER/dsn/2009_v2_no1/postmarketing.htm# Atomoxetine

Faraone SV (2008). Lisdexamfetamine dimesylate: the first long-acting prodrug stimulant treatment for attention deficit/hyperactivity disorder. *Expert Opin Pharmacother* **9**(9): 1565–74.

Faraone SV, Biederman J, Morley CP, Spencer TJ. (2008) Effect of stimulants on height and weight: a review of the literature. *J Am Acad Child Adolesc Psychiatry* **47**(9): 994–1009.

Graham J, Coghill D (2008) Adverse Effects of Pharmacotherapies for Attention-Deficit Hyperactivity Disorder. *Epidemiology, Prevention and Management CNS Drugs* **22**(3): 213–37.

Greenhill L, Kollins L, Abikoff H, McCracken J, Riddle M, Swanson J, McGough J, Wigal S, Wigal T, Vitiello B, Skrobala A, Posner K, Ghuman J, Cunningham C, Davies M, Chuang S, Cooper T (2006). Efficacy and safety of immediate-release methylphenidate treatment for preschoolers with ADHD. *J Am Acad Child Adolesc Psychiatry* **45**(11): 1284–93.

Mannuzza S, Klein RG, Truong NL, Moulton JL 3rd, Roizen ER, Howell KH, Castellanos FX (2008). Age of methylphenidate treatment initiation in children with ADHD and later substance abuse: prospective follow-up into adulthood. *Am J Psychiatry* **165**(5): 604–9.

Mehta MA, Owen AM, Sahakian BJ, Mavaddat N. Pickard JD, Robbins TW (2000). Methylphenidate enhances working memory by modulating discrete frontal and parietal lobe regions in the human brain. *J Neurosci.* **20**(6): RC65.

Michelson D, Buitelaar JK Danckaerts M, Gillberg C, Spencer TJ, Zuddas A, Faries DE, Zhang S, Biederman J (2004). Relapse prevention in pediatric patients with ADHD treated with atomoxetine: a randomized, double-blind, placebo-controlled study. *J Am Acad Child Adolesc Psychiatry* **43**(7): 896–904.

MTA Cooperative group (1999). A 14-month randomized clinical trial of treatment strategies for attention-deficit/hyperactivity disorder. Multimodal Treatment Study of Children with ADHD. *Arch Gen Psychiatry* **56**(12): 1073–86.

National Institute Clinical Excellence (2008). Attention deficit hyperactivity disorder: full guideline. http://www.nice.org.uk:80/nicemedia/pdf/CG72FullGuideline.pdf

Peterson K, McDonagh MS, Fu R. (2008). Comparative benefits and harms of competing medications for adults with attention-deficit hyperactivity disorder: a systematic review and indirect comparison meta-analysis. *Psychopharmacology (Berl)* **197**(1): 1–1.

Sallee F, McGough J, Wigal T, Donahue J, Lyne A, Biederman J (2008); Guanfacine Extended Release in Children and Adolescents with Attention-Deficit/Hyperactivity Disorder: A Placebo-Controlled Trial. *J Am Acad Child Adolesc Psychiatry*. [Epub ahead of print].

Schweitzer JB, Lee DO, Hanford RB, Zink CF, Ely TD, Tagamets MA, Hoffman JM, Grafton ST, Kilts CD (2004) Effect of methylphenidate on executive functioning in adults with ADHD: normalization of behavior but not related brain activity. *Biol Psychiatry* **56**: 597–60.

Scottish Intercollegiate Guidelines Network (SIGN) (2001) Attention deficit and hyperkinetic disorders in children and young people: a national clinical guideline. Vol. 52. Edinburgh.

Swanson CJ, Perry KW, Koch-Krueger S, Katner J, Svensson KA, Bymaster FP (2006). Effect of the attention deficit/hyperactivity disorder drug atomoxetine on extracellular concentrations of norepinephrine and dopamine in several brain regions of the rat. *Neuropharmacology* **50**(6): 755–60.

Swanson JM, Elliott GR, Greenhill LL, Wigal T, Arnold LE, Vitiello B, Hechtman L, Epstein JN, Pelham WE, Abikoff HB, Newcorn JH, Molina BS, Hinshaw SP, Wells KC, Hoza B, Jensen PS, Gibbons RD, Hur K, Stehli A, Davies M, March JS, Conners CK, Caron M, Volkow ND (2007). Effects of stimulant medication on growth rates across 3 years in the MTA follow-up. *J Am Acad Child Adolesc Psychiatry* **46**(8): 1015–27.

Taylor E, Döpfner M, Sergeant J, Asherson P, Banaschewski T, Buitelaar J, Coghill D, Danckaerts M, Rothenberger A, Sonuga-Barke E, Steinhausen HC, Zuddas A (2004). European clinical guidelines for hyperkinetic disorder—first upgrade. *Eur Child Adolesc Psychiatry* **13**(Suppl 1): I7–30.

Torres AR, Whitney J, Gonzalez-Heydrich J (2008). Attention-deficit/hyperactivity disorder in pediatric patients with epilepsy: Review of pharmacological treatment. *Epilepsy & Behavior* **12**: 217–33.

Tourette's Syndrome Study Group (2002). Treatment of ADHD in children with tics: a randomized controlled trial. *Neurology* **26**: 58(4): 527–36.

Volkow ND, Fowler JS, Wang GJ, Telang F, Logan J, Wong C, Ma J, Pradhan K, Benveniste H, Swanson JM (2008). Methylphenidate Decreased the Amount of Glucose Needed by the Brain to Perform a Cognitive Task. *PLoS ONE* **3**(4): e2017.

Wilens TE, Adler LA, Adams J, Sgambati S, Rotrosen J, Sawtelle R, Utzinger L, Fusillo S (2008). Misuse and diversion of stimulants prescribed for ADHD: a systematic review of the literature. *J Am Acad Child Adolesc Psychiatry* **47**(1): 21–31.

Chapter 6

Psychosocial and other non-pharmacological treatments

Manfred Döpfner

Key points

- Psychosocial interventions for children and adolescents with ADHD include
  - psychoeducation of the patient and their parents/ teachers;
  - family based psychosocial interventions, in particular behavioural parent training
  - pre-school, kindergarten and school based psychosocial interventions
  - peer-focused behavioural interventions and social skills training
  - cognitive therapies for the child
- Other non-pharmacological interventions in children and adolescents which have at least some empirical support include neurofeedback and diet
- In adults smaller studies provide some support for coaching and cognitive behavioural interventions, in both individual and group formats that support an individual's self-management strategies.

6.1 Introduction

Psychosocial treatments aim to reduce ADHD-symptoms and other associated behavioural and emotional problems and thus increase the psychosocial functioning of the patient and their quality of life. Well established psychosocial interventions for reducing ADHD symptoms and the other associated disruptive symptoms include psychoeducation of the patient and the parents/teachers, behavioural parent training including family interventions, teacher training, and behavioural classroom management strategies including interventions in pre-school, kindergarten and school as well as peer-focused behavioural interventions with social skills training and cognitive behavioural therapy of the patient (Taylor et al., 2004; Pelham & Fabiano, 2008).

Psychoeducation is the basis of every treatment; however the effects of psychoeducation have not been well evaluated. Behavioural parent training and school based behavioural interventions are empirically the best established psychosocial interventions while the effects of peer-focused behavioural interventions and social skills trainings and cognitive behavioural therapy of the patient have been less well studied. A combination of several of these interventions is often required since each of these interventions has its own particular strengths and treatment objectives. This combined treatment is also often called multimodal psychosocial treatment. Other psychosocial interventions (e.g. psychoanalytically oriented treatment, play therapy, systemic family therapy) have either not been assessed regarding their empirical effects on ADHD symptoms or are not supported in this respect in empirical trials. Several other non-pharmacological interventions (diet, neurofeedback) have at least some support.

Most of the empirical trials for non-pharmacological treatments have been conducted using young children with combined type of ADHD, a few with the primarily inattentive subtype of ADHD, and a few with adolescents or adults with ADHD. The following chapters describe content and empirical support of the different interventions as well as their treatment indications.

6.2 **Psychoeducation**

Psychoeducation for the patient and the parents is the base of any treatment. The main aims of psychoeducation are listed in Box 6.1.

Box 6.1 Aims of psychoeducation

- development of a therapeutic relationship with the patient and the parents
- collection of information about their individual health beliefs and attributions
- based on these health beliefs the information of the patient, the parents (and teachers) about ADHD
- definition of treatment goals as well as the development of a conjoint treatment plan.

In order to assess the individual health beliefs and attributions both the child, their parents, and, if consent is given by the family, the teacher are interviewed. These individual beliefs about causes of the specific problems and their potential solution form the basis for informing the patients and his/her relatives about the evidence-based knowledge of what ADHD is, and for the development of a shared understanding of both the causes of the problem and the therapeutic interventions that are required. The information given should include all main areas of evidence based knowledge about ADHD, especially symptoms, aetiology, course, prognosis, and treatment and should also cover what is not known. The education of children has to be adapted dependent on their level of development. The importance of psychoeducation for the child increases with age. While the education of pre-school children can be difficult according to the stage of their cognitive development psychoeducation should be given to all school-aged children.

Although psychoeducation is seen as a basic tool in the therapy of mental illness there are no studies which evaluate its effects in ADHD. Some indirect support comes from multimodal treatment studies showing symptom reductions during initial psychoeducation and enhanced treatment effects by combining psychoeducation with pharmacotherapy compared to pharmacotherapy alone (e.g. Doepfner *et al.*, 2004).

6.3 **Family-based psychosocial interventions**

Behavioural parent training (BPT) has been shown to be effective in improving the child's behaviour and decreasing maladaptive parental behaviour. In some studies additional positive effects on reducing parental stress and improving child classroom behaviour have also been shown. However the generalization of treatment effects from the family to other situations (e.g. school) is the exception rather than the rule. BPT explicitly provides parents with a range of behaviour modification techniques that are based on social learning principles (see Box 6.2, adapted from Taylor *et al.*, 2004).

Most training programmes last between 8 and 12 sessions. In spite of many differences in design and implementation between different programmes behavioural parent training is one of the most successful psychosocial interventions for the treatment of children with ADHD and it meets the criteria for being a well-established treatment with substantial evidence of efficacy (Pelham & Fabiano, 2008).

> ### Box 6.2 Components of behavioural parent training
>
> Identification of specific problem situations, and specific behaviour problems within these problem situations.
>
> An analysis of positive and negative consequences and contingencies of appropriate and problem behaviours together with the parents.
>
> If coercive and unpleasant parent-child interactions occur very often, while positive parent-child interactions rarely occur, attempts should be made to enhance parental attending skills during supervised playtime sessions.
>
> Teaching the parents effective methods of communicating commands and how to set rules and of pay positive attention to their child's compliance.
>
> The use of token systems in order to reinforce appropriate behaviour in specific situations.
>
> The development together with the parents of *appropriate* mild negative consequences for problem behaviour. These consequences should be closely and consistently linked to the problem behaviour.
>
> Teaching the use of response cost systems in order to reduce very frequent behaviour problems. Parents are taught to remove chips or points from a pool if the problem behaviour occurs. The remaining chips belong to the child and can be changed into backup reinforcers.
>
> Teaching the use of time-out from reinforcement as a punishment procedure for more serious forms of child non-compliance if negative consequences to problem behaviour are not effective. This intervention has to be explained very carefully to the parents and has to be monitored very carefully lest it become punitive.
>
> In adolescence, teaching the use of contingency contracting rather than token systems or response cost systems and stress self management procedures. The use of problem-solving and communication training as well as cognitive restructuring is supported with the aim of reducing parent-adolescent conflicts.

Behavioural parent training has demonstrated positive effects in individual (e.g Sonuga-Barke *et al.*, 2001) as well as group settings (e.g. Pelham, & Hoza, 1996). Positive effects of parent training has been demonstrated for children of all age-groups—for pre-school children at risk for ADHD (Sonuga-Barke *et al.*, 2001, Hautmann *et al.*, 2008) school aged children (Pelham, & Hoza, 1996; Doepfner *et al.*, 2004) and adolescents (McLeary, & Ridley, 1999). Unfortunately little is known about the differential effects of other parent or child characteristics on the outcome of these programmes. Sonuga-Barke, Daley, and Thompson (2002) reported that the presence of maternal ADHD resulted in less child improvement than non-ADHD maternal status when the mother participated in a BPT class, demonstrating a negative moderating effect of parental psychopathology on treatment outcome.

Some but not all studies have shown an additional benefit can be achieved by combining parent training with medication. Firm conclusions about the additional effects of medication on parent training are difficult to draw from most of the studies which combine different interventions especially where studies have included additional interventions on top of the parent training and medication, e.g. additive school interventions or even more complex programmes.

6.4 Psychosocial interventions in pre-school and school settings

The main components of psychosocial interventions delivered in the pre-school and school settings are; the discussion of classroom structure and task demands with the teacher, the identification of specific problem situations and specific behaviour problems, the analysis of positive and negative consequences and contingencies of appropriate and problem behaviours, the enhancement of the differential attending skills of the teacher, and the implementation of token economy systems, response cost systems, and brief time-out from reinforcement. The integration of the child as an active member in this therapeutic process is important (Taylor et al., 2004).

Using a higher level classification classroom intervention can be distinguished from academic intervention.

- **Classroom interventions** include modifications of the classroom itself and strategies of behavioural classroom management.
- **Academic interventions** can be defined as school interventions that focus on promoting conditions conducive to improving academic achievement.

Teaching the teachers about ADHD as well as about treatment strategies (psychoeducation) is important in order to increase the likelihood that the psychosocial interventions are implemented within the school. This also depends on the cooperation of school to creating a setting within which the teacher can actively and willingly take part in the treatment of a child.

Another crucial point for the effective implementation of school based interventions is the establishment of an effective collaboration between the home and the school. Conflicts between the two, which can be instigated by either party, ignoring the work of the other or working on different goals can lead to frustration of the teacher and/or the parents and reduce the effectiveness of the intervention.

6.4.1 **Classroom interventions**
The overall approach to teaching children with ADHD should involve paying attention to the structuring of the whole classroom environment and not only to specific tasks. A common intervention is the use of individual and separated desks to achieve a decrease of distraction. The use of visual aids as posters and signals can also be used to structure the classroom. Studies also show that traditional classroom settings with rows and opposite-sex seating can increase task engagement and lead to lower levels of distractability.

Other well established behavioural classroom management interventions include specific behavioural techniques as praise, planned ignoring, giving effective commands, daily report cards as well as the use of contingency management techniques (e.g. incentives, reward programs, point systems, time-out).

Several reviews and meta-analyses have shown behavioural classroom management to be effective (Chronis et al., 2006; Daly et al., 2007; Fabiano et al., 2009; Pelham, & Fabiano, 2008). Most studies show effects on both classroom behaviour and social adjustment but the effects on academic performance are less clear. Many studies have used single subject designs and only a few have examined the effects of classroom interventions using a between-group design. Miranda (2006) demonstrated the effects of a multi-component classroom intervention which included psychoeducation for the teacher, use of contingency management, instructional management procedures as well as changes in classroom environment and use of self-instructional procedures. This programme resulted in significant improvements in ADHD symptoms, and reduced school problems and antisocial behaviour rated by both parents and teachers.

6.4.2 **Academic interventions**
Although it is well recognized that children with ADHD are at risk for significantly lower academic achievement and poor academic outcomes very little treatment research has been conducted in this area. Peer tutoring, computer assisted instruction, task and instructional modifications and strategy training are all potential interventions that aim to increase on-task behaviour and thus enhance academic achievement.

Peer tutoring is an instructional strategy whereby two students work together on an academic task with one student providing assistance, instruction and feedback to the other. All models of peer tutoring aim at the increase of on-task behaviour and the enhancement of attention. A well described model is the classwide peer tutoring (CWPT; Greenwood et al.,1988). Here tutoring is carried out by tutoring pairs with praise and points for correct answers and correction with subsequent practicing for wrong answers. CWTP has

> **Box 6.3 Recommendations for altering academic tasks (Barkley, 2006)**
>
> - Matching the tasks to each child´s abilities
> - Varying the presentation format and task materials to maintain interest and motivation
> - Brief and one-at-a-time presentation of academic assignments
> - Enthusiastic yet task-focused presentation with the possibility of frequent and active child participation
> - Interspersing academic periods with brief periods of physical exercise
> - Scheduling the more academic subjects into the morning hours
> - Reducing the length of written assignments
> - Allowing extra time for written tests.

been shown to result in increased in active engagement in academic tasks and reduced in off-task behaviour with a subsequent improvement in academic performance by ADHD students (DuPaul *et al.*, 1998).

Another method of academic intervention uses the modification of tasks and instructions. Task modifications involve revision of the curricula, whereas modification of instructions involves adapting the content and delivery of instructions to meet the needs of ADHD children (see Box 6.3).

Again there are only very few studies exploring the effects of task and instructional modification.

A very specific form of instructional modification is the use of computer-assisted instruction (CAI) to improve the academic achievements of students with ADHD. Specific instructional characteristics of CAI include: the highlighting of essential material, the use of multiple sensory modalities, the division of content material into smaller bits of information, the provision of immediate feedback about response accuracy, and limiting the presentation of nonessential and distracting features. The few studies of CAI that have been conducted report an increase in both attention and on task behaviour.

Strategy training is another form of academic intervention and is closely related to the strategies that are taught in cognitive therapy. Strategy training helps the student to develop a set of strategies which are specifically designed to address the demands of an academic situation and which can directly address the students needs, e.g. taking notes or self-reinforcement.

6.5 **Peer interventions and social skills trainings**

Interventions aimed at increasing social skills were developed in an attempt to reduce the social problems which frequently result from the core symptoms of ADHD. These interventions focus on the development and reinforcement of appropriate social skills such as communication, cooperation, participation, and validation. Unfortunately traditional office-based social skills training produces minimal effects and the social validity of these interventions is therefore questionable. Several studies do however support the use of behavioural interventions aimed at reducing peer relationship problems in recreational settings, typically summer treatment programmes. These usually combine social skill training, reward cost system, group practice as well as sport and membership skills. Positive effects including enhanced social functioning have been shown in several randomized controlled studies (Pelham & Fabiano, 2008). In a comparably complex after-school programme for middle scholars, Molina et al. (2008) targeted educational, social and recreational skills, homework completion, and school and home behaviour in a 10-week programme and showed greater improvements in functioning of the active treatment group compared to a comparison group.

6.6 **Cognitive behaviour therapy of the patient**

Cognitive behavioural therapies all aim to promote self-controlled behaviour through the enhancement of problem-solving strategies. Several different types of cognitive behavioural treatments aimed at helping children with ADHD have been developed. These have included a variety of techniques including verbal self-instructions, problem-solving strategies, cognitive modelling, self-monitoring, self-evaluation, and self-reinforcement. Although a lot of research has been conducted using these different types of cognitive-behavioural interventions no clinically important changes have yet been demonstrated on either behavioural measures or academic performance in children with ADHD. There is however some limited evidence that a combination of social skills training and problem-solving interventions can show positive effects if they are combined with intensive, multi-component behavioural treatment packages.

Facilitating core skills of executive functioning is another recent approach. In one study a computerized training of working memory increased both working memory and other neuropsychological skills and reduced maternally rated ADHD symptoms (Klingberg et al., 2005).

6.7 **Multimodal psychosocial interventions**

A multimodal psychosocial treatment approach, utilizing a combination of several of the psychosocial interventions described above, is often needed since children typically present with a variety of problems and each of these interventions focuses on different treatment objectives. It is therefore unsurprising that the majority of clinical trials have included treatment packages that included all or some combination of the behavioural interventions. Outcomes have typically been measured for each domain independently, the suggestion being that the intervention component targeted at a particular domain was responsible for the outcomes in that domain and the conclusion being drawn that all components are necessary to bring about overall change in the child. Although this may be the case in most cases it remains an assumption that is not yet backed by empirical evidence.

In the Multimodal Treatment Study of ADHD (MTA; MTA Study Group, 1999), the "behavioural treatment" package included a course of behavioural parent training along with a school intervention, and a summer programme over the course of a 14-month intervention. With respect to ADHD symptoms, the behavioural treatment group was not significantly different from the community treatment comparison group—a randomly assigned condition receiving treatment as usual from community providers, 68% of whom received medication for ADHD during the treatment period. In addition, and often not reported, at 14 months the behavioural group was superior to the medication management group, who received the MTA medication algorithm, with respect to parent satisfaction with treatment and parent-perceived improvement in referring problems (Pelham et al., 2008), and on observed parenting skills (Wells et al., 2006).

Both the results of the MTA-study and meta-analyses of other trials using psychosocial interventions suggest that in the short-term the effect sizes of psychosocial interventions are roughly about the half that of stimulant medication for ADHD core symptoms. However, despite the superiority of the medication algorithm at the end of the active treatment phase, follow-up observational studies of the MTA groups did not find substantial lasting differential effects of the different treatment modalities in the long-term once the study treatments were withdrawn and the children and their families were free to choose what treatment they received from their local providers (Swanson et al., 2007).

Most of the studies discussed above have been conducted with the patients of children with combined type ADHD. A training that combined teacher consultation, parent training, and child skills training (skills for independence and social competence) was however shown to be effective in reducing symptoms as well as in increasing organisational and social skills in children with predominantly inattentive subtype (Pfiffner et al., 2007).

In view of our current lack of knowledge about which components of a multimodal treatment approach actually make a difference an alternative to combining all the different interventions together at one point of time an alternative approach suggested by the European guidelines (Taylor et al., 2004) and as evaluated in at least one study (Döpfner et al., 2004) whereby a more individually tailored adaptive multimodal treatment approach dependent on the particular problems shown by an individual (stepwise care) may be a good alternative for many children.

6.8 **Neurofeedback**

Neurofeedback, a specialized type of biofeedback, is an operant conditioning procedure that attempts to enhance self-regulation of brain-activity. Over about 25–50 sessions brain electrical activity is recorded by an electroencephalogram (EEG) and immediately fed back to the patient using visual or acoustic signals. Reinforcement is given when the patient changes their brain activity in a certain direction. These changes are supposed to have an impact on behavioural parameters. Neurofeedback for patients with ADHD aims to reduce activity within the theta-band and enhance acitivity in the beta-band. This pattern of brain wave activity is supposed to be related with an attentive but relaxed state and less hyperactive symptoms. A meta-analysis by Riccio and French (2004) showed positive outcomes in 17 of 18 studies for children with ADHD. Unfortunately many of these studies have significant methodological limitations. Despite the growing evidence for neurofeedback as a valuable treatment module in neuropsychiatric disorders further, controlled studies are necessary to establish clinical efficacy and effectiveness and to learn more about the mechanisms underlying successful training.

6.9 **Food additives and restriction diets**

Numerous food additives have been proposed to have a substantial impact on ADHD symptoms but only a few of these have been investigated in randomized-controlled studies.

Essential omega-3 and omega-6 fatty acids are phospholipids which are contained in neuronal cell membranes of the brain. They are supposed to exert a positive effect on neurotransmission and so it has been hypothesized that a lack of those polyunsaturated fatty acids may play a major role in the pathogenesis of ADHD. These fatty acids cannot be synthesized by the human body and therefore have to be obtained from foodstuffs or added as food supplements.

Investigations of the effects of omega-3 and omega-6 fatty acid supplementation have reported inconsistent results. Some studies found no reduction in ADHD-symptoms after docosahexaenoic acid (DHA) supplementation was given to a group of children diagnosed with ADHD while other trials with eicosapentaenoic acid (EPA) or combinations of essential fatty acids which include EPA have been reported to ameliorate ADHD-related symptoms in populations with elevated ADHD symptoms (Richardson & Montgomery, 2005) or in patients with the inattentive subtype of ADHD (Johnson et al., 2008). Most of these studies have several methodological limitations. A sensible conclusion at this point in time would appear to be that these treatments are still in an experimental phase.

Some food components have been postulated to have a negative impact on behaviour and it has been supposed that the elimination or restriction of those components from the diets of children with ADHD will decrease ADHD-symptoms. Such substances include sugar, several preservatives, food colourings, and potentially allergenic foodstuffs. In the main evidence for their effects on ADHD symptoms is rather weak and for sugars there is considerable evidence that it does not result in hyperactivity. The intake of a mixture of sodium benzoate preservatives and several artificial additives did however result in increased ADHD symptoms in 3- and 8/9-year-old children in a double blind trial conducted in a general population sample (McCann et al., 2007). However further studies are needed to address the question whether restricting these additives in the diets of children with ADHD will reduce their symptoms.

6.10 **Non-pharmacological treatment options for adults with ADHD**

In recent years there has been growing awareness for the need for non-pharmacological treatment options for adults with ADHD of which 20 and 50% do not show significant symptom reduction with medication or are unable to tolerate ADHD medications. And even those who do respond to medication often have only symptom reductions of 50% or less. Also, adults requesting treatment for ADHD usually have complex problems extending well beyond the core ADHD symptoms which are unlikely to respond to ADHD medication.

Non-pharmacological treatments for adults with ADHD include counselling, coaching and individual or group cognitive-behavioural therapy. Unfortunately these approached have received very little in the way of research investigation.

Counselling and psychoeducation can be conducted in either an individual or a group setting and has considerable conceptual overlap with cognitive-behaviour therapy. Patients receive information about ADHD and are taught strategies to meet their individual goals. Although there are workbooks to support this approach (Weiss, 1994) no studies have investigated the effects of these counselling approaches on adults with ADHD.

Coaching is defined as a supportive and pragmatic process. The patient and their personal coach work together, usually via short daily telephone calls, with the aim of identifying goals and to developing strategies to meet them (Barkley, 2006). To date there is no standard methodology and no research has been done on this form of intervention for adults with ADHD.

Research on cognitive-behaviour therapy for adults with ADHD is also still in its infancy. There are however some small studies investigating the effects of group and individual CBT using Linehan's Dialectical Behavioral Therapy approach (Hesslinger *et al.*, 2002), brief cognitive-behavioural interventions that focus on psychoeducation, comorbid symptoms and self-esteem, in both group and individual settings that have shown some positive effects. Because of small sample sizes and only few randomised controlled trials effects must be regarded as tentative. Further research is desperately needed, particularly concerning the differential effects of medication and CBT.

References

Barkley, R (2006). Attention-Deficid Hyperactivity Disorder: *A Handbook for diagnosis and treatment* (3rd ed.). New York: Guilford.

Chronis, AM, Jones, HA, & Raggi, VL (2006). Evidence-based psychosocial treatments for children and adolescents with attention-deficit/ hyperactivity disorder. *Clinical Psychology Review* **26**: 486–502.

Daly, BP, Creed, T, Xanthopoulos, M, & Brown, RT (2007). Psychosocial Treatments for Children with Attention Deficit/Hyperactivity Disorder. *Neuropsychology Review* **17**: 73–89.

Doepfner, M, Breuer, D, Schurmann, S, Metternich, TW, Rademacher, C & Lehmkuhl, G (2004). Effectiveness of an adaptive multimodal treatment in children with Attention-Deficit Hyperactivity Disorder—global outcome. *European Child and Adolescent Psychiatry* **13** Suppl 1: 117–29.

DuPaul, G J, Ervin, R A, Hook, CL, & McGoey, KE (1998). Peer tutoring for children with attention deficit hyperacitivity disorder: Effects on classroom behavior and academic performance. *Journal of Applied Behavior Analysis* **31**: 579–92.

Fabiano, GA, Pelham, WE, Coles, EK, Gnagy, EM, Chronis-Tuscano, A & O'Connor, BC (2009). A meta-analysis of behavioral treatments for attention-deficit/hyperactivity disorder. *Clinical Psychology Review* **29**: 129–40.

Greenwood, CR, Delquadri, J, & Carta, JJ (1988). *Classwide peer tutoring.* Seattle: Educational Achievement Systems.

Hautmann, C, Hanisch, C, Mayer, I, Plück, J & Döpfner, M (2008). Effectiveness of the prevention program for externalizing problem behaviour (PEP) in children with symptoms of attention-deficit/hyperactivity disorder and oppositional defiant disorder—generalization to the real world. *Journal of Neural Transmission* **115**(2): 363–70.

Hesslinger, B, Tebartz van Eltst, L, Nyberg, E, Dykierek, P, Richter, H, Berner, M & Ebert, D (2002). Psychotherapy of attention deficit hyperactivity disorder in adults: A pilot study using a structured skills training program. *European Archives of Psychiatry and Clinical Neuroscience* **252**:177–84.

Johnson, M, Östlund, S, Fransson, G., Kadesjö, B, & Gillberg, C (2008). Omega-3/Omega-6 Fatty Acids for Attention Deficit Hyperactivity Disorder. A Randomized Placebo-Controlled Trial in Children and Adolescents. *Journal of Attention Disorders OnlineFirst*, doi:10.1177/1087054708316261.

Klingberg, T, Fernell, E, Olesen, PJ, Johnson, M, Gustafsson, P, Dahlstrom, K, Gillberg, CG, Forssberg, H & Westerberg, H (2005). Computerized training of working memory in children with ADHD—a randomized, controlled trial. *J Am Acad Child Adolesc Psychiatry* **44**(2): 177–86.

McCann, D, Barrett, A, Cooper, C, Crumpler, D, Dalen, L, Grimshaw, K, Kitchin, E, Lok, K, Porteous, L, Prince, E, Sonuga-Barke, E, O'Warner, J, & Stevenson, J (2007). Food additives and hyperactive behaviour in 3-year-old and 8/9-year-old children in the community a randomized, double-blinded, placebo-controlled trial. *Lancet* **370**: 1560–7.

McLeary, L, & Ridley, T (1999). Parenting adolescents with ADHD: Evaluation of a psychoeducation group. *Patient Education and Counseling* **38**: 3–10.

Miranda, A, Jarque, S, & Rosel, J (2006). Treatment of children with ADHD: psychopedagogical program at school versus psychostimulant medication. *Psicothema* **18**: 335–41.

Molina, BGG, Flory, K, Bukstein, OG, Greiner, AR, Baker, JL, Krug, V, & Evans, SW (2008). Feasibility and Preliminary Efficacy of an After-School Program for Middle Schoolers With ADHD. *Journal of Attention Disorders Online First*, doi:10.11771087054707311666.

MTA Study Group (1999). A 14-month randomized clinical trial of treatment strategies for attention-deficit/hyperactivity disorder. The MTA Cooperative Group. Multimodal Treatment Study of Children with ADHD. *Archives of General Psychiatry* **56**(12): 1073–86.

Pelham, WE, & Fabiano, GA (2008). Evidence-Based Psychosocial Treatments for Attention-Deficit/Hyperactivity Disorder. *Journal of Clinical Child & Adolescent Psychology* **37**: 184–214.

Pelham, WE & Hoza, B (1996). Intensive treatment: A summer treatment program for children with ADHD. In E Hibbs & P Jensen (Eds), *Psychosocial treatments for child and adolescent disorders: Empirically based strategies for clinical practice.* (pp. 311–40). New York: APA.

Pelham, WE, Wheeler, T, & Chronis, A (1998). Empirically Supported Psychosocial Treatments for Attention Deficit Hyperactivity Disorder. *Journal of Clinical Child Psychology* **27**: 190–205.

Pfiffner, LJ, Mikami, AY, Huang-Pollock, C, Easterlin, B, Zalecki & McBurnett, K (2007). A Randomized, Controlled Trial of Integrated Home-School Behavioural Treatment for ADHD, Predominatnly Inattentive Type. *J Am Acad Child Adolesc Phychiatry* **46**: 1041–50.

Riccio, CA, & French, CL (2004). The status of empirical support for treatment of attention deficits. The Clinical Neuropsychologist 18: 528–58.

Richardson, AJ & Montgomery, P (2005). The Oxford Durham study: A randomized, controlled trial of dietary supplemetation with fatty acids in children with developmental coordination disorder. *Pediatrics* **115**: 1360–6.

Sonuga-Barke, EJS, Daley, D, Thompson, M, Laver-Bradbury, C & Weeks, A (2001). Parent-based therapies for preschool attention-deficit hyperactivity disorder: A randomized, controlled trial with a community sample. *J Am Acad Child Adolesc Phychiatry* **40**: 402–8.

Sonuga-Barke, EJ, Daley, D & Thompson, M (2002). Does maternal ADHD reduce the effectiveness of parent training for preschool children's ADHD? *J Am Acad Child Adolesc Psychiatry* **41**(6): 696–702.

Swanson, JM, Hinshaw, SP, Arnold, LE, Gibbons, RD, Marcus, S, Hur, K, Jensen, PS, Vitiello, B, Abikoff, HB, Greenhill, LL, Hechtman, L, Pelham, WE, Wells, KC, Conners, CK, March, JS, Elliott, GR, Epstein, JN, Hoagwood, K, Hoza, B, Molina, BS, Newcorn, JH, Severe, JB & Wigal, T (2007). Secondary Evaluations of MTA 36-Month Outcomes: Propensity Score and Growth Mixture Model Analyses. *J Am Acad Child Adolesc Psychiatry* **46**(8): 1003–14.

Taylor, E, Döpfner, M, Sergeant, J, Asherson, P, Banaschewski, T, Buitelaar, J, Coghill, D, Danckaerts, M, Rothenberger, A, Sonuga-Barke, E, Steinhausen, H-C, & Zuddas, A.(2004). European clinical guidelined for hyperkinetic disorder—first upgrade. *European Child and Adolescent Psychiatry* (Suppl. 1) **13**: I/7–I/30.

Wells, KC, Chi, TC, Hinshaw, SP, Epstein, JN, Pfiffner, L, Nebel-Schwalm, M, Owens, EB, Arnold, LE, Abikoff, HB, Conners, CK, Elliott, GR, Greenhill, LL, Hechtman, L, Hoza, B, Jensen, PS, March, J, Newcorn, JH, Pelham, WE, Severe, JB, Swanson, J, Vitiello, B & Wigal, T (2006). Treatment-related changes in objectively measured parenting behaviors in the multimodal treatment study of children with attention-deficit/hyperactivity disorder. *J Consult Clin Psychol* **74**(4): 649–57.

Weiss, L (1994). *The attention deficit disorder in adults workbook*. Dallas, Texas: Taylor Publishing Company.

Chapter 7

Organizing and delivering treatment

David Coghill and Marina Danckaerts

Key points

- The delivery of treatment for ADHD can be broken down into several steps
  - Deciding on the targets for treatment
  - Choosing, starting and optimizing the first treatment
  - Monitoring treatment
  - Adjusting and switching treatments
- Treatment is about more than just symptom reduction, it also involves managing comorbid disorders and improving quality of life
- The decision about whether to use a behavioural or pharmacological treatment as the first option is a complex one which depends on a range of different factors
- It is essential to take baseline measures and to continue to monitor both positive and negative outcomes on a regular basis
- When initiating medication treatments for ADHD the use of recognized titration protocols can help to ensure that treatment is optimized
- Similarly the use of a structured protocol for adjusting doses and switching medication will help ensure that evidence based treatment decisions are made whenever possible.

7.1 Introduction

Following diagnosis all children with ADHD will require some form of intervention and most will require treatment over a relatively prolonged period of time. Psychoeducation forms the cornerstone of treatment and should be offered to all of those receiving a diagnosis and their families. Additional treatments are usually indicated and as described in the preceding chapters there are now a broad range of therapeutic approaches available to manage the core ADHD symptoms of which the behavioural psychotherapies and medications are supported by the strongest evidence base. Many children will also require treatment for a range of other psychiatric and non-psychiatric disorders and other coexisting problems such as peer relationship and family difficulties. The material contained in this Chapter will draw heavily on work conducted by the European ADHD Guidelines Group, and will attempt to present a clearly described operationalized version of the evidence based guidance and strategies for initiation, monitoring and maintenance of ADHD treatment previously developed and published by this group (Taylor *et al.* 2004, Banaschewski *et al.* 2006).

The four main sections will deal with; deciding on the targets for treatment, initiating the first ADHD treatment, monitoring treatment, and adjusting and switching treatments. In each section we will make use of "process diagrams" similar to those used in Chapter 4 (see Box 4.1 for a description). As before each of these details the tasks that have to be addressed at each stage of the clinical process. These process diagrams should not be seen as prescriptive and we suggest that they are used to stimulate discussion within teams and services and to help problem solve any barriers to practice and to develop an evidence based care pathway that works for their particular circumstances.

7.2 **Deciding on the targets for treatment**

Most children with ADHD will present with multiple problems in addition to their core ADHD symptoms and the associated impairments. This means that it is usually necessary to decide which problem or problems should be tackled first. Sometimes the decision is simple e.g. child protection concerns clearly outweigh most other problems, but in most circumstances the choice depends on a combination of severity (actual and perceived), relative importance (to the child, their parents, the school and the clinician), the availability of an evidence based treatment and pragmatic clinical decision making (e.g. poor peer relationships and academic functioning with low self esteem are often adjudged to be secondary to ADHD symptoms in which case it would seem sensible to treat the ADHD symptoms first and observe the impact of this on the other difficulties). Whilst it is of course possible to address several problems at the same time it is helpful if, when making a treatment plan one is explicit about what one is and is not hoping to change in order that patient and parent expectations are managed. Making treatment targets explicit also helps set treatment goals and make accurate baseline measures so that treatment change can be monitored adequately with appropriate measures. Broad domains are described in Box 7.1. Within each of these domains it is then necessary to make specific, explicit, clear, achievable targets.

> **Box 7.1 Potential target symptoms and problems**
> - Core ADHD symptoms
> - Oppositional and disruptive behaviour in the home
> - Oppositional and disruptive behaviour in the classroom
> - Academic problems
> - Parent-child relationship and communication problems
> - Peer relationships
> - Other associated symptoms (e.g. anxiety, mood instability, depression, dyspraxia, specific learning disorders, speech, and language problems etc.).

In clinical practice several situations where a child/young person is suffering from more than one psychiatric disorder can present particularly difficult choices. This includes ADHD with comorbid depression, anxiety, Tourette's/tics, pervasive developmental disorder, or substance misuse. These situations are discussed in more detail in section 7.3.

7.3 **Initiating the first ADHD treatment**

7.3.1 **Choosing the correct first treatment**

When the decision is made to start treatment for ADHD, and after psychoeducation is given to the child and its family, it is necessary to consider which treatment should be initiated first (see Box 7.2). There are two main choices to be made at this stage behavioural treatment (usually group parent training) or medication. There have traditionally been differences in the choices made at this stage by European and US clinicians. In the US medication is usually considered to be the first line treatment for all ADHD irrespective of severity. European clinicians have traditionally been more conservative and have reserved medication for those meeting the much more restrictive ICD-10 criteria for hyperkinetic disorder. Recently attitudes across Europe have changed and there has been an increase in the willingness to consider medication for children with less severe ADHD. Recent evidence has provided a degree of support for both views. Santosh *et al.* (2005) reanalyzed data from the influential Multimodal Treatment of ADHD study (MTA study) and found that whilst for children with ICD-10 defined hyperkinetic disorder ("severe pervasive disabling ADHD") a carefully crafted medication management was clearly more effective than an intensive behavioural programme, for those with less severe ADHD there was little difference between the two approaches. On the basis of these results the European ADHD Guidelines group have recommended that medication should be considered as a first line treatment for children with hyperkinetic disorder—unless of course there are any contraindications to medication. Either medication or behavioural treatment (usually in the form of group parent training and/or school based behaviour modification programmes) can be considered as the initial treatment for those with less severe ADHD (Taylor *et al.*, 2004) with the implication that behavioural treatment will usually, but not always, be the most appropriate first option. In the UK, the National Institute for Health and Clinical Excellence (NICE, 2008) has taken a similar, although maybe less flexible, approach and recommends that medication, as a first line treatment, should be restricted to those with severe ADHD and that

Box 7.2 Choosing the correct first treatment	
Trigger	• Child/young person is diagnosed with ADHD and decision to treat ADHD symptoms is made
Clinicians involved	• Child and Adolescent Mental Health Services • Developmental/behavioural paediatrics
Aims	• To choose the most appropriate initial treatment
European Guidelines Recommendations	• All of those diagnosed with ADHD (and their families) should receive psychoeducation • Services that diagnose ADHD need to be able to offer/access a wide range of treatments (pharmacological and non-pharmacological) • When the diagnosis is one of ICD-10 hyperkinetic disorder ("severe pervasive and impairing ADHD") the first line treatment is usually medication unless there are contrain-dications to medication • In those with less severe ADHD (DSM-IV ADHD—including inattentive type—but not hyperkinetic disorder) either behavioural treatment or medication can be considered • Additional problems (e.g. reduced social compliance, poor self esteem and family stress) will also usually need to be addressed and will require a broad range of therapeutic skills • Comorbid disorders e.g. specific learning disorders (dyslexia), dyspraxia and other psychiatric disorders may necessitate alternations to the treatment plan or additional treatment.
Outcomes	• Initial treatment choices are made using evidence based principles

group parent-training/education programme, either on its own or together with a group treatment programme for the child should be offered to all and should be the first treatment for those with less severe ADHD. On balance we feel that the European Guidelines Group recommendations are appropriate in most circumstances. There are of course situations where behavioural treatment is not practical. For example mental illness, substance misuse, language barriers or poverty in parents may all make behavioural treatment unfeasible. There are situations where rapid change is required and this is more likely to occur with medication. Also, some families will choose medication over behavioural treatments.

7.3.2 Choosing the first medication

There are now several medications and several formulations licensed for the treatment of ADHD (see Chapter 5 for a review). It is therefore important to think about the general order in which these should be considered and under which circumstances these general rules should be broken. These questions were recently addressed in detail by the European Guidelines Group (Banaschewski *et al.*, 2006). They decided that, on the basis of the available evidence, in most cases methylphenidate will be the first choice medication. Atomoxetine may however be considered as first choice under particular circumstances such as:

- a current or past history of substance misuse
- in the presence of tics
- in the presence of anxiety
- where there is a strong family preference to avoid stimulants
- where 24 hour duration of action is particularly strongly required.

They also considered whether the immediate or extended release stimulant preparations are to be preferred as first line treatments and concluded that, where cost is important and a stimulant is being thought of, an immediate release preparation will usually be the first choice. However an extended release stimulant may be considered important to reduce stigma and increase privacy, where compliance needs to be addressed and to reduce the chance of diversion. Which extended release preparation is chosen will depend on the desired profile of action required across the day.

95

7.3.2.1 *Special circumstances*

As noted in Chapter 2 when ADHD occurs in association with other disorders alteration to the treatment plan is sometimes required. The following recommendations take into account the available evidence.

ADHD + Depression

The clinician should determine which disorder requires to be addressed first. If it is the depression that is causing the most severe impairments and concern, then usual treatment guidelines for depression should be followed after which the ADHD symptoms can be addressed following the principles outlined above. Where the ADHD is to be treated first stimulant medication, if required, should be titrated carefully as this may further lower mood. Otherwise treatment should follow the usual pathway with secondary treatments being offered for depression should this not resolve with treatment of the ADHD. The potential for drug x drug interactions should be remembered. This is particularly relevant for atomoxetine and fluoxetine both of which are metabolised by CYP 4D6 and co-prescription can lead to increased levels of both drugs.

ADHD + Anxiety

ADHD with comorbid anxiety disorders is not necessarily refractory to stimulants and anxiety is not a contraindication. There is some evidence to suggest that atomoxetine may reduce anxiety symptoms in the presence of ADHD and it may therefore be considered in such cases. However, a further search for psychological stresses on the child is always in order, and if they cannot be simply alleviated then psychological treatment may have more to offer than repeated drug trials.

ADHD + Tics

Comorbid tics may sometimes be worsened by stimulants. This is not inevitable, and stimulants are sometimes useful even for the hyperactivity seen in Tourette's syndrome. Atomoxetine is an alternative and appears to be less likely to exacerbate tics. Where atomoxetine is ineffective and methylphenidate whilst effective is exacerbating tics (and a dosage reduction does not lead to an improvement), or if the tics are continuing to cause significant psychosocial impairment, the use of a tic-reducing medication either as a monotherapy or in parallel with ADHD medication (e.g. tiapride, risperidone, sulpiride, clonidine) seems to be indicated. Behavioural therapy may be added for tics and obsessive symptoms.

ADHD + Pervasive Developmental disorder

It is always appropriate for these cases to be seen by specialist services. There is little trial evidence, but we suggest that even in autism it may be worth trying a trial of medication for the symptoms of ADHD although these should be started at the lowest practical dose and titrated slowly and carefully as these children are more likely to suffer from adverse effects even at low doses. Methylphenidate itself is often the most helpful; clonidine, atomoxetine, and even risperidone may have their place. Behavioural therapy, targeting the ADHD symptoms, is also widely applicable.

ADHD + Substance Misuse

There is little research evidence to guide clinicians when treating individuals with ADHD and an established substance misuse disorder, Treatment plans should address both disorders and should include psychosocial interventions aimed at reducing substance misuse and relapse prevention. There are indications that effective treatment of core ADHD symptoms may enhance effective treatment of substance misuse. Pharmacological therapies for ADHD should be started with caution and under close supervision. Atomoxetine is unlikely to be abused and extended release stimulants are likely to be less abusable than their immediate release counterparts.

7.3.3 **Initiating a new medication**

Clinical trials have shown that ADHD medications are very effective at reducing core symptoms and that in many cases both symptoms and impairment can be reduced such that impairment is minimal. This does however require the child to be treated with the right medication at optimal doses (see Box 7.3). Not every patient will respond to every medication and, for the stimulants at least, it is not possible to predict the most effective dose from consideration of the patient's age or weight or the severity of their symptoms. It is therefore necessary to titrate patients onto each new medication whilst carefully measuring both their response to medication and any adverse effects (See Chapter 4).

Key to this process is the routine use of standardized rating scales to measure treatment response and the routine assessment of adverse effects.

There are a wide range of available measures for assessing treatment response. In our clinic we favour the SNAP rating scale (Swanson *et al.*, 2005) used as a clinician rated semi-structured interview with parents and patient. The ADHD and oppositional defiant disorders section are used at each appointment as we find that giving the parents a chance to discuss their child's oppositionality often helps them give a clearer and less prejudicial account of the ADHD symptoms. Parent and teacher ratings, using the 10 item Connors' questionnaires, are also collected at each appointment. It is also helpful to rate global impressions using the Clinical Global Impressions Severity and Improvement scales (CGI-I and CGI-S, NIMH, 1985) and the Children's Global Assessment Scale (CGAS, Shaffer, 1983) which are both quick and reliable ways of monitoring overall improvement.

For adverse effects it is helpful to have a standardized set of questions to rate the presence or absence of common adverse effects and to note whether or not these are impairing. Pulse, blood pressure, height and weight should be measured and charted against age and gender matched norms see Chapter 5 Boxes 5.3 and 5.4).

It is essential that all of these measures are commenced at baseline, *prior* to the first dose of medication, in order that change can be assessed accurately. This is especially important for potential adverse effects as many children with ADHD will have issues with sleep, mood dysregulation, irritability, etc. prior to treatment and this needs to be taken into account when assessing potential adverse effects of treatment.

Box 7.3 Initiating a new medication	
Trigger	• A decision is made to initiate ADHD medication for the first time
Clinicians Involved	• Child and Adolescent Mental Health Services • Developmental/behavioural paediatrics
Aims	• An effective treatment should result in "considerable improvement with no problematic adverse effects" • To stabilize on the most effective dose with the least adverse effects
European Guidelines Recommendations	• Titration protocols should be used to ensure that patient is stablilized on the most effective dose • The use of reliable standardised rating scales (e.g. ADHD-IV rating scale, SNAP, Conners' rating scales) for monitoring treatment effects • Baseline measures should include documentation of levels/presence of both symptoms and potential adverse effects, including; • Pulse and blood pressure—6 monthly • Height and weight (plotted on growth chart) • Appetite, tics, depression, irritability, withdrawal, spontaneity, perservation
Outcomes	• Patient is either stabilised on an effective and tolerable dose of medication or identified as a non-responder (either by virtue of "non-response" or intolerable adverse effects)

7.3.3.1 *Titrating on to methylphenidate*

There are several different protocols for titrating on to methylphenidate. Perhaps the most common is the *forced dose titration* method
whereby the child is started on a low dose (e.g. 5mg of immediate
release bd or tds, or the equivalent of an extended release preparation). Baseline measures are recorded and the child is reviewed after
approximately one week (either in person or by telephone) and baseline measures are repeated. Additional information from school is
obtained using a standardized rating scale if possible. If the child has
improved, and there is no room for further improvement treatment is
continued at the current dose. If there is either improvement with
room for further improvement or no improvement, *and* there are no
significant adverse effects, the dose is increased (e.g. to 10 mg immediate release) and the patient is reviewed a week later. Titration is continued either until there is no further room for improvement (remission), there are significant adverse effects, or the maximum routine
dose is reached (usually 20 mg tds immediate release or 15 mg tds in
children < 25kg). The aim is to get maximum response, with minimum
adverse effects, at the minimum required dose. The European Guidelines recommend a maximum daily dose of around 100 mg (note:
above normal licensed dose) methylphenidate but doses higher than 60
mg are normally only recommended where this is already a clear, but
sub-optimal, response to the 60 mg dose. Thus at the end of the 4
week titration period the clinician will have decided that the patient:

- has responded best to a particular dose
- has responded but cannot tolerate the optimal dose due to
  adverse effects and either
  - shows an acceptable response, with no or tolerable adverse
    effects at a lower dose or
  - does not show an acceptable response at a lower dose
- has not responded at any dose.

Whilst we find this practice is acceptable to most families an alternative
strategy that is less intensive and may be more practical in some situations is for parents to give 5mg of immediate release methylphenidate
on a weekend/holiday morning and then to introduce a cognitively
demanding task about 1 hour later, and observe general effect. If there
are no adverse effects 10 mg can be given on another weekend/holiday
morning (and 15 mg on another in teenagers). Parents draw conclusions as to tolerability and likely effect. If this is favourable they can
discuss with the prescriber extending the trial to mornings only during
school week with the teacher measuring effect with a standardized
rating scale. Where effectiveness is established it is still necessary to
optimize dose and again one should aim for maximum response, with
minimal adverse effects at the minimum dose. It is important to

remember that some adverse common effects such as loss of appetite or sleep problems can sometimes be managed by adjusting routines or the timing of doses.

7.3.3.2 *Titrating on to dexamfetamine*

Clinicians titrating patients on to dexamfetamine can follow the same procedures described for methylphenidate but with reduced doses (5mg methylphenidate ≈ 2.5mg dexamfetamine).

7.3.3.3 *Titrating on to atomoxetine*

As atomoxetine is prescribed in a mg/kg fashion, it is generally simpler to titrate than the stimulants. The standard protocol for titration on to atomoxetine is to initiate treatment at a dose of 0.5 mg/kg to reduce difficulties with initial adverse effects (especially nausea which we inform patients is very common but usually transient), increasing to 1.2 mg/kg after 1 week and then continued at this dose. Most of those who are going to show a response will report some positive effects after 3–4 weeks, however in our clinical experience there is a small group of patients who, whilst showing no response at around 8 weeks do report significant benefits at around 12 weeks. We therefore recommend that patients are made aware of this and that treatment is continued for 12 weeks before a decision about non-response is made. If there is a response to 1.2 mg/kg but there remains room for improvement it is acceptable to increase the dose up to 1.8 mg/kg.

7.4 **Monitoring treatment**

Having established and stabilized effective treatment it is necessary to put systems in place to monitor ongoing treatment (see Box 7.4). Whilst a proportion of patients will probably continue to do well with minimal intervention many will require more careful monitoring either to ensure continued clinical response or to minimize the impact of adverse effects such as the sleep and appetite difficulties common with stimulants. Others will require additional support and/or treatment for other types of problem such as mood lability, peer and family relationship difficulties, etc. The results of the MTA study suggested that a carefully crafted and applied medication management system is superior to that which was traditionally available in the community. Group treated under MTA medication management protocol:

- were treated with doses 10 mg/day greater
- had 3-times–daily dosing versus twice-daily dosing
- started treatment with intensive 28 day double blind titration trial
- received more in the way of supportive counselling and reading materials
- had their dosage adjustments informed by monthly teacher consultation with the pharmacotherapist.

Box 7.4 Monitoring treatment	
Trigger	• Child/young person has been stabilized on a treatment regime
Clinicians involved	• Child and Adolescent Mental Health Services • Developmental/behavioural paediatrics • Primary care staff

Aims	• To monitor the impact of treatment
	  • To ensure treatment is still required
	  • To ensure that treatment results in an adequate continued response without problematic adverse effects
	• To identify non-responders, relapers and those with new or as yet untreated problems

European Guidelines Recommendations	• A regular (at least 6 monthly), and as required, review supervised by a specialist (who may be working with primary care staff in a shared care setting)
	• The continued use of reliable standardised rating scales (eg. ADHD-IV rating scales, SNAP, Conners' rating scales) and/or specific treatment targets are helpful for monitoring treatment effects
	• If on medication measures should include documentation of levels/presence of both symptoms and potential adverse effects, including:
	  • Pulse and blood pressure (ECG not routinely required unless there are specific cardiac risk fators)—6 monthly
	  • Height and weight (plotted on grownth chart)—6 monthly
	  • Appetite, tics, depression, irritability, withdrawal, spontaneity, perseveration—each visit

Outcomes	• Nobody on treatment that they don't require • The majority of those on treatment will be optimally controlled with no problematic adverse effects • Those who require a switch of treatment or additional treatment are identified

101

The routine follow up of treatment response and adverse effects is important and should be given adequate time and consideration. It is important to get feedback from teachers and young people as well as parents. This can help achieve optimal symptom control and avoid anomalous situations arising such as a rather high dose of medication being arrived at from parent feedback before the message gets through that teachers are concerned about undue subduing of the child. It is not necessary for senior clinical staff to conduct all continuing care clinics. Indeed if a well thought through protocol is designed and implemented it is possible for junior medical staff and nurses to conduct high quality continuing care clinics. The same protocol, assessment schedule and measurement tools can be used for continuing care clinics as were used when initiating and titrating on to medication.

Although rarely made explicit the key aim of most clinical care is to improve quality of life. Various studies have identified that ADHD severely impairs a person's quality of life and evidence is emerging that treating ADHD can relieve at least some of this burdon (Danckaerts *et al.*, in press). Although to date mainly used in a research setting several validated measures of quality of life are now available to the clinician at relatively little cost (e.g. PEDS-QL and CHIP-CE). More widespread use within routine clinical practice can help to ensure that the clinician is focusing on the whole picture and not just on core symptoms.

It is good practice to routinely and regularly ensure that an individual continues to require medication. With stimulants it is generally recommended that an individual has a planned withdrawal from medication at least once a year in order to assess whether symptoms return. In reality this will usually occur naturally and in an unplanned fashion when a patient forgets to take their medication and others around them either notice the difference or will comment that there seemed to be no difference between days when medication was taken and when it was missed. A continued need for medication is more difficult to demonstrate with atomoxetine in view of its different mechanism of action and in particular because it has a more long-term pharmacodynamic effect. If a short withdrawal of atomoxetine results in a recurrence of symptoms them one can conclude it should be restarted. If however symptoms do not immediately return after a short term withdrawal it is still possible that they will return after a longer break. In itself this situation does not raise any problems as we can withdraw medication and wait to see if symptoms return. The problem for many families is that if symptoms do return after a moderate to long withdrawal it is possible that it will take time to get another appointment at the clinic and that even when atomoxetine is restarted it may take several weeks for the symptoms to resolve again. During this time the patient will continue to have difficulties that they and their family, understandably, will see as having been avoidable. There is no simple solution to this situation other than to ensure that withdrawal is monitored closely and that the patient has quick and easy access to the clinic if required.

It is essential to remember that the management of ADHD involves a lot more than just the management of the core ADHD symptoms. Comorbidity is very common as are other personal, interpersonal and systemic issues. These will often require treatment in their own right. It is not uncommon for clinicians and patients/parents to be working to different agendas at a continuing care clinic with the clinician for example wanting to discuss the response of ADHD symptoms to medication and the parents wishing to discuss other issues such as problems they are having interfacing with school or their child's peer relationships etc.. For this reason we have found it helpful to be clear that the dual purpose of the routine continuing care clinic is to monitor treatment and *identify* "other problems". Separate appointments are then made to ensure that these "other problems" are managed in the most appropriate manner by the most appropriate person and that adequate time is devoted to each stage of the clinical process.

Although around one third of those with ADHD no longer suffer from impairments in adulthood many young people continue to have significant symptoms of ADHD or have other coexisting conditions that continue to require treatment past the normal cut-off age for paediatric and child and adolescent mental health services. For these individuals it is therefore very important to consider their ongoing treatment requirements and make arrangement for their care to be passed on to the appropriate adult services (see section 5.7.3). Usually this will be to adult psychiatry. It is important that time is taken to ensure that there is a smooth transition between services and that all relevant details of the past and anticipated future treatment and services that the young person will require are passed on. It is often helpful for there to be a formal meeting involving the child and adolescent mental health service and/or paediatrics and the adult psychiatric services to discuss the handover of care. Clearly the young person, should be involved in the planning and where appropriate, so should their parents or carers.

The precise timing of transition will vary locally but should usually be completed by the time the young person is 18 years old.

7.5 Adjusting and switching treatment

Where there is a failure to respond to a particular treatment or when a patient is unable to tolerate a treatment due to adverse effects it is necessary to consider either adjusting or switching treatment. In general, although the need for change may have been recognized within primary care, such alterations to the treatment plan should usually be carried out by specialists within child and mental health services or paediatrics. Particularly in the case of suspected non-response there are several general considerations that need to be addressed in all cases before deciding on what action to take. These include reviewing dosage (always ensure and adequate dose has been applied before switching treatment), addressing compliance issues (motivational interviewing may help compliance, if on an immediate release preparation try an extended release one) and diagnosis and assessing whether the apparent non-response is actually due to a coexisting problem that is not currently being treated.

When the lack of response is due to intolerable adverse effects or is indicative of the patient being resistant to that particular form of treatment the recommendations for switching treatments vary depending on the current and past treatment history.

The responses to various situations requiring a switch of treatment are described in Table 7.1.

7.6 **I want to implement evidence based practice in my clinic but am not sure how to get started**

Chapters 4 and 7 of this book provide a framework for developing and evidence based protocol for assessing and managing ADHD based on the European ADHD Guidelines (Taylor *et al.*, 2004, Banaschewski *et al.*, 2006). Whilst translating evidence into routine clinical practice is never easy it is possible. It requires dedication, willingness to critically self reflect, a team that work together as a unit and who are willing to embrace change. And whilst it does require time and resources it does not necessarily require either a significant investment of money or huge numbers of staff. and it can be very satisfying to practice in the knowledge that you are doing all that you can to ensure each patient receives the right treatment at the right time.

It is not possible to describe a recipe for change that will work in every setting. ADHD care is delivered in very diverse settings each with its own history and barriers to change, and within a wide range of health care systems that require the clinician to organize their care in very different ways.

Table 7.1 Switching treatments	
Current treatment	**Suggested interventions**
Mild to moderate ADHD either unable to adhere to, or failing to respond to, a first line behavioural intervention (after a trial of around 2 months)	Initiate a trial of methylphenidate
Failure to respond to methylphenidate as a first line treatment	Ensure dose has been optimized
	Address any compliance issues
	Switch to either dexamfetamine or atomoxetine
Methylphenidate not tolerated as a first line treatment	Switch to atomoxetine
Failure to respond to atomoxetine as a first line treatment	Ensure dose has been optimized and that treatment has continued for long enough (~ 12 weeks)
	Address any compliance issues
	Switch to either methylphenidate or dexamfetamine
Atomoxetine not tolerated as a first line treatment	Switch to either methylphenidate or dexamfetamine
Failure to respond to (or tolerate) methylphenidate, dexamfetamine and atomoxetine	Seek advice from regional/national specialist
	Try alternative medications; • Bupropion • Tricyclic antidepressant • Alpha 2 agonist (clonidine, guanfacine) • Mood stabilizer • Nicotine patch

Note; these recommendations will continue to change as new treatments, drugs/ preparations become available, it is therefore important that the clinician stays up to date with new advances in the field.

However it is possible to present some general guidelines that will facilitate the development of evidence based care pathways. One effective strategy is to address the need for change with a problem solving approach and utilize the concepts of clinical audit to monitor and inform cycles of change. Possible steps are outlined in Box 7.5.

Box 7.5 A problem solving approach to implementing evidence based practice

Agree on standards of practice to be followed (local, national, international evidence based guidelines)

Measure current practice against these standards

- This could be against the complete guidelines or only particular sections.
- Could be done by a single clinic or a group of services

Identify where practice is adequate and where improvements need to be made to achieve the agreed standards

Identify the current barriers to implementing these standards of care

Spend time as a team problem solving and identifying the steps required to overcome these barriers and achieve implementation of evidence based practice in your workplace

Implement agreed changes

Reassess practice against the standards

Continue with this process until the team are happy that practice meets standards (both your own and those set out in guidelines)

References

Banaschewski , Coghill D, Santosh P et al. (2006) Long-acting medications for the hyperkinetic disorders. A systematic review and European treatment guideline. *Eur.Child Adolesc.Psychiatry* **15**(8): 476–45.

Danckaerts M, Sonuga-Barke EJS, Banaschewski T et al. The Quality of Life of Children with Attention Deficit/Hyperactivity Disorder: A Systematic Review. *Eur.Child Adolesc.Psychiatry* In Press.

National Institute for Mental Health. Clinical Global Impressions. (1985) *Psychopharmacol.Bull.* **21**(4) 839–43.

Santosh PJ, Taylor E, Swanson J et al. (2005) Refining the diagnoses of inattention and overactivity syndromes: A reanalysis of the Multimodal Treatment study of attention deficit hyperactivity disorder (ADHD) based on ICD-10 criteria for hyperkinetic disorder. *Clinical Neuroscience Research* **5**(5–6): 307–14.

Shaffer D, Gould MS, Brasic J et al. (1983) A children's global assessment scale (CGAS). *Arch.Gen.Psychiatry* **40**(11): 1228–1231.

Swanson J, Schuck S, Mann M, Carlson C, Hartman K, Sergeant J, et al. (2005). Categorical and dimensional definitions and evaluations of symptoms of ADHD: The SNAP and the SWAN Ratings Scales [Draft]. Available at: http://www.adhd.net/SNAP_SWAN.pdf. Accessed May 25, 2005.

Taylor E, Dopfner M, Sergeant J et al. (2004) European clinical guidelines for hyperkinetic disorder—first upgrade. *Eur.Child Adolesc.Psychiatry* **13** Suppl 1: I7–30.

Appendix

This appendix contains addresses and links to ADHD self-helping organizations which might be useful for the reader. The authors do not guarantee the accuracy, relevance, timeliness, or completeness of this information. Further, the inclusion of addresses of and links to particular organizations does not guarantee their quality or importance, nor do the authors intend to endorse any views expressed, or services offered, of these organizations or on their websites.

Global Networks

AD/HD Global Network
North America, P.O. Box 3700, Mc Allen TX 78502, USA
South America, Colonia 1767 apt. 11, Montevideo 11200, Uruguay
Europe, Ben-Gurion Drive 161, 60437 Frankfurt, Germany
Australia, P.O. Box 204, Chatswood 2057 NSW, Australia
E-mail: info@global-adhd.org
Website: www.global-adhd.org

ADHD-Europe
Website: www.adhdeurope.eu

Latin American League for ADHD
Website: tdahlatinoamerica.org

National Networks
Argentina

La Fundacion Trastorno Por Deficit de Atención e Hiperactividad, Ernestina Montefusco de Pergolini, Castelli 313, Drive 4, Code Postal 1704 Bunches Mejía Prov. Bs.As., Tel Fax: (011) 4658-1515
Email: tdah@tdah.org.ar
Website: www.tdah.org.ar

Australia

Canberra and Queanbeyan ADD Support Group Inc, PO Box 717, Mawson ACT 2620, Tel: 02 6290 1984 bh—02 6287 4608
Email: info@addact.org.au
Website: www.addact.org.au

Austria

ADAPT—Aufmerksamkeitsdefizit/Hyperaktivitaetsstoerungen—
Arbeitsgruppe zur Foerderung von Personen mit AD/HS und
Teilleistungsschwaechen, Landstrasse Hauptstrasse 84, 1030 Vienna,
Austria, Tel 0676–516 56 87 (mobile), Fax +43 1 879 75 48
Email: verein_adapt@yahoo.com
Website: http://www.adapt.at

Belgium

Association "Hyperactivité et troubles associés—TDA/H Belgique",
Rue du Châtelain, 19 Boite 4-1000 Bruxelles, Tel: 0484 177 708
Email: tdah.be@coditel.net
Website: www.tdah.be/

Zit Stil, 321, Heistraat, B-2610 Wilrijk, Tel 03/8303025,
Fax: 03/8252072
Website: www.zitstil.be/zitstil/

Bolivia

Fundación para Educación y Servicio, Grupo DIA Cochabamba
Bolivia; Tel. & Fax.: 00591 444240539
Email: gabrielahirmas@yahoo.com
Website: www.adders.org/boliviamap.htm

Brazil

Brazilian Association of ADHD, Prof. Paulo Mattos
Website: www.tdah.org.br/

Puerto Alegre ADHD outpatient Program (PRODAH)
Website: www6.ufrgs.br/prodah/

Rua Sen Pinheiro Machado 80/402 J Amália 1, Volta Redonda—
RJ Brazil, Sandra de Jesus Travassos, Tel: (+55 24) 344-6323—
Fax (+5524) 344-4699
E-mail: travassos@csn.com.br
Website: www.adders.org/brazilmap.htm

Canada

AD/HD Foundation of Canada, 11 Florence Street, Ottawa, Ontario,
K2P 0W6, Tel: (613) 233-2343
Email: info@adhdfoundation.ca
Website: www.adhdfoundation.ca

Canadian ADHD Resource Alliance (CADDRA), 40 Wynford Drive,
Suite 304A, Toronto, Ontario, M3C 1J5
Website: www.caddra.ca

CADDAC—Centre for ADD/ADHD Advocacy, Canada
40 Wynford Drive, Suite 304B, Toronto, Ontario, M3C 1J5, Canada
tel: 416-637-8584, fax: 416-385-3232
E-mail: info@caddac.ca

Columbia
Fundación GRADAS, Carrera 35, No. 8A-38 Local 3, Medellín
http://www.gradas.org.co/

Costa Rica
Fundación DA, Apartado 232-2300, San José

Croatia
Awakening—Association for Understanding ADHD, Zagreb, Croatia
phone: +385 98 997 8915
E-mail: info@hyperactivedreamers.com
Website: www.hyperactivedreamers.com

Cyprus
ADD-ADHD Support, P.O. Box 12187, 2341 Nicosia,
Tel: +357-22446592, Mb: +357-99651995, Fax:+357-22446593
Email: sue@add-adhd.org.cy
Website: www.add-adhd.org.cy/

Denmark
The DAMP Association, Kongensgade 68, 2., DK-5000 Odense C
Tel. +45 7021 5055, Fax +45 7021 5055
E-mail: info@damp.dk
Website: www.adders.org/denmarkmap.htm

ADHD-foreningen
Website: www.adhd.dk

Estonia
Email: info@elf.ee
Website: www.elf.ee

Finland
Suomen MBD-liittory/The Finnish association for ADHD, ADD and
MBD, Sitratie 7, Fin-00420 Helsinki, Tel. : + 358-9-454 111 20,
Fax: + 358-9-454 111 23
Email: adhd@adhd-liitto.fi
Website: http://www.adhd-liitto.fi

Association for Adults with ADHD in Finland, Suomen
AD/HD—Aikuiset ry, c/o Ritva Kohijoki, Lepistöntie 5, 05400 Jokela,
040-521 2645 (ACN)
Email: sihteeri@adhd-aikuiset.org
Website: www.adhd-aikuiset.org

France

Association « HyperSupers—TDAH France, 2 sentier de la fontaine
77160 PROVINS, Tel. : +336 19 30 12 10
E-mail: info@TDAH-France.org
Website: www.TDAH-France.org

Germany

Website: www.zentrales-adhs-netz.de

ADHS Deutschland e.V., Poschingerstraße 16, 12157 Berlin, Postfach
41 07 24, 12117 Berlin, Tel.: 030-85 60 59 02, Fax: 030-85 60 59 70
E-Mail: info@adhs-deutschland.de

Bundesvereinigung Aufmerksamkeitsstörung Deutschland e. V.,
Obergraben 25, 56567 Neuwied, Tel.: 0 26 31–5 46 41
E-Mail: info@juvemus.de
Website: www.bv-ad.de

Gibraltar

Email: Giselle addersgibraltar@yahoo.com

Greece

E-mail: kouki@otenet. kouki@otenet.gr
website: http://www.childmentalhealth.gr/
Website: www.specialeducation.gr/
Website: www.parents.gr/

Great Britain

National Attention Deficit Disorder Information and Support
Service —ADDISS, PO Box 340, Edgware, Middlesex HA8 9HL,
Tel.: 020 8952 2800, Fax: 020 8952 2909
E-mail: info@addiss.co.uk
Website: www.addiss.co.uk

Hong Kong

ADD Adult Support Group, Therapy Associates Limited,
12/F California Tower, 21 D'Aguilar St., Central, Hong Kong,
Tel.: 2869-1962
Website: www.talhk.com/topics/add.htm

Hungary

Website: www.adhd-magyarorszag.com/.

Iceland

ADHD Association in Iceland, Háaleitisbraut 13, 108 Reykjavík,
Iceland, Tel: +354-581-1110
Email: adhd@adhd.is
Website: www.adhd.is/

India

AIKYA, 1/1,Bhagirathi Ammal Street, R.A.Puram, Chennai 600 028.
Tel: 91-44-493 8443 / 91-44-499 3892
Email: aikyaschool@hotmail.com or parvathyv@hotmail.com

Ireland

Irish National Council of AD/HD Support Groups is an umbrella
organisation for the AD/HD Support Groups active throughout the
country
WebSite: www.incadds.ie/support-groups.php

Hadd Family Support Group, Carmichael Centre For Voluntary
Groups, Carmichael House, North Brunswick Street, Dublin 7
Tel:01 8748349
Email: info@hadd.ie

Israel

Herzliyya; 20 Ha 'Shahafim Street, Ra'Anana 43724; Judith Schwarcz,
Tel: 09-7729888, Fax: 09-7729889, Mobile: 052-488288
Email: moogy@netvision.net.il

Lisa Grossman; Pardess Meshutaf 5, Raanana: Tel: 09-7729253
Email: grossmanld@012.net.il
Website: www.lisagrossman.com

Italy

Associazione Italiana Famiglie ADHD, Napoli, Viale Colli
Aminei 60-80131 Napoli or Rignano Flaminio (Roma),
Via Montaroni 27, Tel 0761.508126, Fax 06-233227628
E-mail: segreteria@aifa.it
Website: www.aifa.it/

Associazione Italiana Disturbi Attenzione e Iperattività, Bergamo, Via
Locatelli 62, Tel (+39) 035 223012
E-mail: aidai@libero.it
website: www.aidaiassociazione.com

Italian National ADHD Registry
A description (in Italian) of the Italian National ADHD Registry with
information for parents and clinician can be found at the Italian
National Institute of Health (Instituto Superiore di Sanità-ISS)
E-mail: adhd@iss.it
Website: www.iss.it/adhd/

Japan

NPO Edison Club, Ms. Keiko Takayama, 924, 1-1-1, Toyooka,
Iruma-Shi, Saitama, 358-0003, Japan FAX; +81-4-2962-8683,
E-mail: info@e-club.jp
Website: www.e-club.jp (only Japanese)

Luxembourg

Spontan ADD a.s.b.l. , Boîte Postale 5, L-8001 Strassen, 26 25 95 95
E-mail: help@adhs.lu
Website: www.adhs.lu/spontan/index.php

Malaysia

Family Support Group for ADHD/LD and related disorders
Website: groups.yahoo.com/group/myadhdsupport/

Malta

The ADHD Family Support Group, P.O. Box No. 2, St. Julians STJ
1001, Malta, Tel: 00356 21 233 749 (Ans.Mach)
Email: info@adhdmalta.org
Website: www.adhdmalta.org

Mexico

Adriana Pérez de Legaspi, Directora, Asociación Mexicana por el
Déficit de Atención, Hiperactividad y Trastornos Asociados A.C
E-mail: hiperactividad@exatec.itesm.mx
Website: www.deficitdeatencion.org

Netherlands

Impuls—Vereniging voor volwassenen met ADHD en aanverwante
stoornissen, Postbus 93, 3720 AB Bilthoven, Tel.: (030) 225 50 50,
Fax: (030) 225 24 40
Email: info@impulsdigitaal.nl.
Website: www.impulsdigitaal.nl

New Zealand

ADHD.org.nz, C/O ADDvocate NZ Inc., P.O Box 249,
Tauranga, New Zealand
E-mail: addvocate@xtra.co.nz
Website: www.adhd.org.nz

Norway
The Norway Association for MBD/ ADHD
Website: www.mbd.no

Peru
Asociación Peruana de Déficit de Atención
Website: www.deficitdeatencionperu.org/

Philippines
Website: www.adders.org/404.html

Poland
Polish ADHD Association (in Polish: Polskie Towarzystwo ADHD)
ul. Siewna 10, 31-230 Kraków (Kracow), Tel/Fax: +48 122 514 924
Email: ptadhd@ptadhd.pl
Website: www.ptadhd.pl/

Puerto Rico
Dorado CH.A.D.D., Calle 5, bloque 3 #3CC, Doraville, Dorado,
Puerto Rico 00646
Website: expage.com/page/doradochadd

Romania
Societatea Româna Speranta, Strada Fagului Numarul 17Cod postal
1900 Temisoara, Tel 0040 256 190 245, Fax 0040 256 201 152
Email: societatearomanasperanta@yahoo.com
Website: www.intermeding.com/speranta/

Saudi Arabia
ADHD Support Group and ADHD Society, Neurosciences
Department MBC 76, King Faisal Specialist Hospital and Research
Centre, Kingdom of Saudi Arabia, P.O Box 3354 Riyadh 11211,
Tel: +966-1-442-4981, Fax: +966-1-442-3435
Website: www.adhd.org.sa
Email: adhdarabia@hotmail.com

Singapore
SPARK, 75 Sophia Road, Singapore 228156, Bella Chin, President
Email: chinbella@hotmail.com
Website: http://www.spark.org.sg

South Africa
Attention Deficit and Hyperactivity Association of South Africa
(ADHASA)
Website: www.adhdsupport.co.za

113

ADHD Support Group, P.O. Box 3704, Randburg 2125, Republic of
South Africa, Tel: (011) 888-7655
Email: rscox@icon.co.za or marinavzyl@yahoo.com

Spain

ADANA Fundación (Ayuda Déficit de Atención, Niños,
Adolescentes y Adultos) Barcelona, Isabel Rubio,
Calle Muntaner 250, principal 1°, Barcelona, 08021, Spain,
Tel. 93. 24119 79 Fax. 93 24119 77
E-mall: adana@gcelsa.com
http://www.f-adana.org/

Federación Española de Asociaciones de Ayuda al Déficit de
Atención e Hiperactividad, Colegio San Carlos, C/Del Romeral, n° 8,
Tentegorra, 30205 Cartagena Murcia
E-mail: adahimurcia@hotmail.com/penchom@cesmurcia.es
Website: www.feaadah.org

Sweden

Riksförbundet Attention, Förmanvägen 2, 117 43 Stockholm
Website: www.attention-riks.se/

Switzerland

Verein für Eltern und Bezugspersonen von Kindern sowie für
Erwachsene mit POS/AD(H)S, Elpos Schweiz, Sekretariat, Postfach
255, 3047 Bremgarten
E-mail: info@elpos.ch
Website: www.elpos.ch

Fachgesellschaft für Aufmerksamkeitsdefizit/Hyperaktivitätsstörung
3047 Bremgarten b. Bern, Schweiz
E-mail: sekretariat@sfg-adhs.ch
Website: www.sfg-adhs.ch

USA

CHADD National Office, 8181 Professional Place—Suite 150,
Landover, MD 20785, Tel: 001-301-306-7070 / Fax: 001-301-306-7090
Website: www.chadd.org

Attention Deficit Disorder Association, PO Box 7557, Wilmington,
DE 19803-9997, Tel./Fax: (800) 939-1019
Email: adda@jmoadmin.com
Website: www.add.org

Index

A

academic interventions 81, 82–83
ADHD
  comorbid profile 10f
  definition of 3
  symptoms of 3–6, 49t
ADHD Rating Scale (ADHD-RS) 36t
adult ADHD
  non-pharmacological treatments for 87–88
  pharmacological treatments for 73–74
  prevalence of 7
  prognosis, course and outcome of 14–15
adverse effects
  of atomoxetine 67
  of medication 97–98
  of stimulants 62, 65–66
amitriptyline 70
amfetamine 54, 55–57, 58f, 64, 72
anxiety disorders 10, 37t, 96
appetite loss 62
assessment 34–40, 42–49
  clinical interview with the parents 44–45
  clinical procedures 34–40
  diagnosis and formulation 48, 49t
  intelligence and cognitive testing 47–48
  interview schedules 34–35
  interview with the child 45–46
  neuropsychological assessments 38
  observations 36–37, 46–47
  physical evaluation and investigations 47, 48t
  process of 40–49
  questionnaires 35–36
  recognition of ADHD, 41–42
  telephone interview with teachers 47
atomoxetine 25, 53, 54, 65, 71, 73, 74, 95, 96, 97, 105t
  adverse effects of 67
  clinical efficacy 61–63
  interactions with other drugs 60
  mechanism of action 55, 56f
  pharmacokinetics of 59–60
  precautions during treatment 69
  relapse prevention by 64
  titration on to 100
  treatment monitoring 101
Attention-Deficit/Hyperactivity Disorder. see ADHD
autism 11, 73, 96

B

Behavioural Assessment System for Children (BASC) 36t
behavioural parent training (BPT) 78, 79–81
behavioural therapy 84, 88, 96
biofeedback 86
bipolar disorder 10–11, 66
blood pressure 66
boys, prevalence of ADHD in 12–13
brain function and neuropsychology 26–29
brain, structure of the 24
broad band questionnaires 35, 36t
bupropion 70, 105t

C

CAPA interview 35t
cardiovascular effects, of ADHD medication 67–69
Child and Adolescent Psychiatric Assessment (CAPA) 35t
Child Behaviour Checklist (CBCL) 35, 36t
Child Depression Inventory (CDI) 37t
Children's Communication Checklist 37t
Children's Global Assessment Scale 97
Children's Manifest Anxiety Scale, Revised (R-CMAS) 37t
Children's Sleep Habits Questionnaire (CSHQ) 37t
Children's Social Behaviour Questionnaire (CSBQ) 37t
classroom interventions 81, 82
classwide peer tutoring 82–83
clinical assessment. See assessment
Clinical Global Impressions Severity and Improvement scales 97
clinical presentation 8
clomipramine 70
clonidine 59, 69–70, 96, 105t
coaching 88
cognitive behavioural therapy 78, 84, 87, 88
cognitive impairments 27–28
comorbid diagnoses 9
comorbid disorders 9–12
  bipolar disorder 10–11
  conduct disorder 9
  developmental coordination disorder 12
  emotional disorders 10
  language delays 11–12
  learning disorders 11–12
  neuropsychological deficits 12
  oppositional defiant disorder 9
  pervasive developmental disorders 11
  sleep problems 12
  substance abuse 11
  tic disorders 11
computer-assisted instruction (CAI) 83
Concerta XL®, 58, 74
conduct disorder 9
Conners Parent Rating Scales - Revised (CPRS-R) 36t
Conners Teacher Rating Scales - Revised (CTRS-R) 36t
coordination disorders 37t
counselling 25t, 87–8
course of ADHD 13–15

D

DAWBA interview 34, 35t
delay aversion 29
depression 37t, 96
desipramine 70, 71
Development and Well-being Assessment (DAWBA) 34, 35t

developmental coordination disorder 12
Developmental Coordination Disorder Questionnaire (DCD-Q) 37t
dexamfetamine 53, 54, 56f, 57, 66, 100, 105t
diagnosis
  of ADHD, 3, 5, 8
  and formulation 48, 49t
  of HKD 3
Diagnostic Interview for Children and Adolescents (DICA) 35t
Diagnostic Interview Schedule for Children (DISC) 34, 35t
diet, restriction 86–7
differential diagnoses 8–9
3,4-dihydroxyphenylethylene glycol (DHPG) 59
docosahexaenoic acid 87
dopamine 20, 21, 24, 25, 26, 54, 55, 56f, 64, 70
DSM-IV 3, 4, 5, 6, 7
dyscalculia 37t
dyslexia 37t
dyspraxia 37t

E

effect sizes 61
eicosapentaenoic acid 87
emotional disorders 10
environmental factors 21–3, 25
  genetic and 23–4
  post-natal environment 22–3
  pre-natal factors 21–2
epidemiology 7
epilepsy 66
Equasym XL® 58, 74
etiology 20–4
  clinical implications of current understanding of 25t
  environmental factors 21–3
  gene-environmental interplay 23–4
  genetics 20–1
EUNETHYDIS, 2
evidence based practice, implementation of 104–5, 106t
executive dysfunctions 27, 29

F

family-based psychosocial interventions 79–81
florid psychosis 66
fluoxetine 60, 96

food additives 86–7
forced dose titration method 99
functional imaging studies 28f

G

gender, and ADHD, 12–13
genetic counselling 25t
genetics
  and ADHD 20–1
  interaction between environment and 23–4, 30f
girls, prevalence of ADHD, 12–13
growth dysregulation 65
guanfacine 70, 105t

H

HKD (hyperkinetic disorder) 93
  definition 3
  ICD-10 criteria for 5, 6
  symptoms 4
hyperactivity 4, 5
Hyperkinetic Conduct Disorder 6

I

ICD-10 3, 4, 5, 6, 7
imipramine 70, 71
impulsivity 4, 5
inattention 4, 5
insomnia 62, 66
instruction modifications 83
intelligence and cognitive testing 47–8
interview schedules 34–5
  semi-structured clinical interviews 34
  structured interviews 34

K

K-SADS-PL interview 35t

L

language delays 11–12, 37t
learning disorders 11–12, 37t
lisdesamfetamine 57

M

mania 37t, 66
medications
  for ADHD and anxiety disorders 96
  for ADHD and depression 96

for ADHD and PDD, 96
for ADHD and substance abuse 97
for ADHD and tics 96
choosing the first medication 95–7
initiation of new 97–100
titration on to atomoxetine 100
titration on to dexamfetamine 100
titration on to methylphenidate 99–100
Medikinet Retard®, 58, 74
methylphenidate (MPH) 25, 53, 54, 69, 72, 95, 96, 105t
  adverse effects of 65, 66
  cardiovascular effects of 67, 68
  extended release preparations 57–9
  interactions with other drugs 59
  mechanism of action 55, 56f
  pharmacokinetics of 57–9
  plasma levels 58f
  safety 64
  titration on to 99–100
modafinil 72
modification of tasks and instructions 83
monitoring of treatment 100–3
multimodal psychosocial interventions 78, 85–6
Multimodal Treatment Study of ADHD, 85

N

narrow band questionnaires 35, 36t
neurochemistry 25–6
neurofeedback 86
neuropsychological assessments 38, 39f, 39t, 40t
non-pharmacological treatments 77–90
  for adults with ADHD, 87–8
  cognitive behavioural therapy 84
  family-based psychosocial interventions 79–81
  food additives and restriction diets 86–7
  multimodal psychosocial interventions 85–6
  neurofeedback 86
  peer interventions and social skills training 84
  psychoeducation 78–9
  psychosocial interventions 81–3

norepinephrine 20, 25, 54, 55, 56f, 59, 70, 71
normalization rates 61
nortriptyline 70, 71
Number Needed to Treat (NNT) 61

O

observations 36–7, 39t, 46–7
Obsessive Compulsive Disorder 37t
omega-3 fatty acid 86–7
omega-6 fatty acid 86–7
oppositional defiant disorder 9
outcomes of ADHD, 13–15

P

PACS interview 34, 35
parent and teacher ratings 97
parent training 78, 79–81
Parent version of the Young Mania Rating Scale (P-YMRS) 37t
Parental Account of Children's Symptoms (PACS) 35t
parenting 23
parents, clinical interview with 44–5
paroxetine 60
pathophysiology 24–9
  brain function and neuro-psychology 26–9
  brain structure 24
  neurochemistry 25–6
  subtypes 29
peer interventions 84
peer tutoring 82
peri-natal factors 22
pervasive developmental disorders (PDD) 11, 37t, 73, 96
pharmacological treatments 53–76
  in adults 73–4
  in children with autism of pervasive development disorders (PDD) 73
  clinical efficacy 60–4
  interactions with other drugs 55–60
  molecular mechanisms of 56f
  precautions before starting medications 68
  precautions during treatment 69
  in preschool children 72–3
  safety 64–9
  severe cardiovascular effects of 67–9
  short term efficacy 60–3

phenytoin 59
phenobarbital 59
physical evaluation and investigations 47, 48t
pimozide 96
post-natal environment 22–3, 25t
potential differential diagnoses 9
pre-natal factors 21–2, 25t
precautions before starting medications 68
precautions during treatment 69
preschool children
  pharmacological treatments 72–3
  prognosis, course and outcome of ADHD 13
  psychosocial interventions 81–3
prevalence of ADHD and HKD, 7
primidone 59
problem-solving strategies 84
process diagrams 40
prognosis of ADHD 13–15
psychoeducation 77, 78–9, 87–8, 91
psychosocial treatments 77–8
  family-based 79–81
  multimodal psychosocial interventions 85–6
  in pre-school and school settings 81–3
pulse rate 66

Q

questionnaires 35–6, 37t
  broad band 35, 36t
  narrow band 35, 36t

R

recognition of ADHD 41–2
relapses, prevention by atomoxetine 64
restriction diets 86–7
risperidone 96
Ritalin LA® 58, 74

S

safety, of pharmacological treatments 64–9
Schedule for Affective Disorders and Schizophrenia for School-Age Children (K-SADS-PL) 35t
schools, psychosocial interventions 81–3

seizures and epilepsy 66
serotonin 20, 24, 26, 54, 70
SKAMP (Swanson, Kotkin, Atkins, McFlynn & Pelham Scale) 36
sleep problems 12, 37t
SNAP rating scale 36t, 97
Social Communication Questionnaire (SCQ) 37t
social skills training 84
state dependence and cognitive impairments 27–8
state regulation deficits 28
Steve-Johnson's syndrome 72
stimulants 95
  adverse effects of 62, 65–6
  efficacy 60–1
  long-term efficacy and efficacy of combination with psychosocial intervention 63
  and substance abuse 64–5
strategy training 83
Strengths and Difficulties Questionnaire (SDQ) 36t
Strengths and Weaknesses of ADHD—Symptoms and Normal Behavior (SWAN) questionnaire 36t
substance abuse 11, 97
  stimulants and 64–5
SWAN questionnaire 36t
symptoms
  of ADHD and HKD, 4
  and problems 49t, 93t

T

task modifications 83
Teacher Rating Form (TRF) 36t
teachers, telephone interview with 35, 47
Test of Word Reading Efficiency (TOWRE) 37t
tiapride 96
tic disorders 11, 37t, 62, 66
  ADHD and 96
Tourette's Disorder Scales—Clinician Rated 37t
Tourette's syndrome 11, 37t, 66, 96
treatment
  adjustment and switching of 103–4, 105t
  choosing the correct first treatment 93–5

deciding on targets for 92–3
initiating the first ADHD, 93–100
monitoring of 100–3
organizing and delivering 91–106
treatment plan 53–4
tricyclics 70–2, 105t

W

weight gain 65
weight loss 62
withdrawal from medication 101
Woodcock-Johnson III questionnaire 37t

Y

Yale-Brown Obsessive Compulsive Scale (Y-BOCS) 37t
Yale Global Tic Severity Scale 37t